Dr. Zalar's book is both a beautiful love story and a chilling tale of the ravages of Alzheimer's disease. Zalar's commitment to his wife throughout her long decline is inspirational and moving. This story should serve as a lesson to us all. Cherish every day with your loved ones because you never know when those days will end—or how.
—Cindy Wojdyla Cain
Joliet Herald News

Doctor Richard Zalar and Trude become more and more real as *Day Is Ending* evolves from its opening on a dreary, and tragic December 7, 1941 to December 7, 2000, the day of Trude's death. This romance is so moving and meaningful because in many ways it is about those "normal" life events that are common to most of us: the first kiss, the roller coaster of courtship, the proposal, marriage, new life, growth, joy, success—and then, a shadow, an inkling, a doubt that insidiously grows into a heartbreaking tragedy. There is no facile resolution offered here. Dr. Zalar simply asks if he would ever have been able to appreciate the depth of this love affair with Trude if they had been spared the torment of Alzheimer's disease. "Why was this allowed to happen?"
—Tom Pamilla, MSW, Director of Programs
Alzheimer's Association, San Diego Chapter

Day is Ending is a remarkably well-recalled story of Dick's and Trude's love, from beginnings to "endings." Their published story may very well serve to lend support to the many dear caregivers of Alzheimer's patients-showing them they are not alone in feeling afraid and/or helpless in their situations. The hands of caregivers are God's hands. Furthermore, Dick's and Trude's love story will certainly be an important revelation to people who have no personal experience with the Alzheimer's disease.
—Garland McCowan Cramer
Friend, who helped bring Trude and Dick together

This is a very moving story about a very personal perspective. I hope others can learn from it the courage needed to face this disease.
—John Trojanowski, M.D., PhD
The Center for Neurodegenerative Research
University of Pennsylvania, Philadelphia

Day
Is
Ending

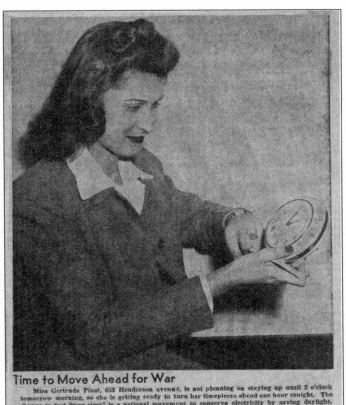

Time to Move Ahead for War
Miss Gertrude Pisut, 653 Henderson avenue, is not planning on staying up until 2 o'clock tomorrow morning, so she is getting ready to turn her timepieces ahead one hour tonight. The change to fast "war time" is a national movement to conserve electricity by saving daylight. (Herald-News photo.)

Day Is Ending

A doctor's love shattered by Alzheimer's disease.

By Richard W. Zalar M.D.

And Walter G. Meyer

C&W Press

C&W Press,
1807 South Washington Street Suite 106
Naperville, IL 60565-2446

www.dayisending.com
email: info@dayisending.com

Printed in the United States of America

ISBN: 0-974-0558-0-8

Library of Congress PCN: 2003104361

Foreword

I found Dr. Zalar's book immensely moving, as well as illuminating. Alzheimer's disease affects many people at a time when life expectancy is growing because so many other once-terminal diseases have been overcome by medical science. Alzheimer's, alas, is not one of them. The more reason to know about it, to understand it, to accept it. Alzheimer's does not, repeat not, overcome the bonds of love and pity, as well as humor and pleasure, between sufferer and caregiver. Love cannot be overcome. Alzheimer's only strengthens it.

JOHN BAYLEY
Author of *Elegy for Iris*
St. Catherine's College
Oxford, England
May, 2002

At the end of what is necessary,
I have come to a place where there is no road.

DAME IRIS MURDOCH
from her novel *Jackson's Dilemma*

Prologue

There were times when I found myself thinking the unthinkable. It would be so easy to end her life. Just a syringe full of morphine. A few grains should be enough. As a physician, I'd have no trouble obtaining that much. Half a grain was enough to deaden pain in a 200 pound man, so three grains should be enough to end the life of a frail, 90-pound, 78-year-old woman.

Or morphine patches might be easier. She had used one before as a pre-scribed pain remedy, containing probably one-half grain. If I just applied five or six of those, they would deaden the central nervous system to the point that her heart and respiration would slow until she just fell into a deeper and deeper sleep from which she would never wake up. It would not be a bad way to go. No resistance, just drowsiness followed by sleep.

But would I want to have to face the consequences afterwards? Perhaps we should go together. I could sedate her, carry her to the garage, put her in the car, get in beside her and start the engine. I could put on one of my favorite cassettes as the exhaust started to fill the garage. It was said that the fumes made you sleepy quickly. I could just fall asleep in the car with her beside me, listening to Tommy Dorsey playing while Jo Stafford sang.

I should leave a note for the housekeeper. I wouldn't want her to find us the next morning with our skins tinged pink from the carbon monoxide.

And I should leave a note for the children. Our son, also a doctor, had strongly hinted that it might be better if his mother died. At times my daughter had also wished her mother dead. But would they forgive me if I took her life and my own? Would it matter after I was gone?

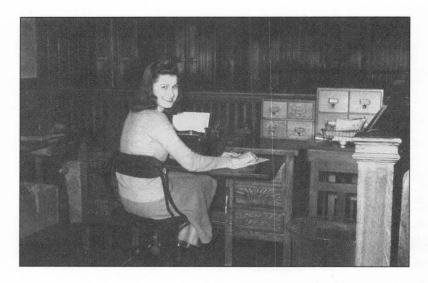

Trude working at her job at
Joliet Township High School.
(top)

Trude Pisut, 1940. (right)

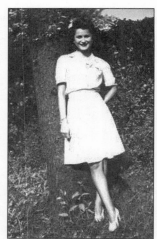

A Girl Named Trude

December 7, 1941 was gray and overcast. That Sunday afternoon I was at my desk in my room at the SAE fraternity house on Daniels Street, doing homework for my classes the next day at the University of Illinois at Champaign-Urbana.

As usual, I was studying with my radio on and had put down my biology notes to tap my pen along to one of my favorite songs. I was quite annoyed when the music suddenly stopped. I can still remember every detail of that day. When a moment happens that changes your life forever, it's hard to forget. It wasn't until another December 7, many years later, that I would experience a date that would change my life as profoundly.

It was about half past noon when the announcer broke into the music to say something to the effect that, "It has just been reported that Japanese planes have attacked the US naval facilities at Pearl Harbor in Hawaii. The attack is still in progress and more details will follow. Stay tuned to NBC for further developments."

Within minutes, Daniels Street in front of the frat house was filled with a mob of students. Many were brandishing their ROTC-issue rifles, waving flags or shouting anti-Japanese slogans. The things people were yelling would be seen as horribly racist now, but back then we didn't even think of terms like "racist." I stayed in my room, too shaken about what this all meant and eager to hear more details to want to join in the frenzied mob assembling on campus.

The next morning many students, especially those in the ROTC program, joined the active military. Just over a year earlier, around my eighteenth birthday, I had registered for the draft, as was required of all young men at that time. Because I was pre-med, I had been placed in the Medical Administration Corps, on inactive status until needed. The war that many saw coming was now upon us and I wasn't sure if my status would change immediately. I wondered if they now needed fighting men more than they could afford to wait for me to become a doctor. My eyesight was poor so the chance of my going into combat was small, but I worried that I could be called up to fill some support role and that my studies would have to be put on hold indefinitely.

As my good friend Russ Stevens put it so succinctly once, "The war ruined everything." Whatever plans any of us had made for our lives were torn up and we faced the blank sheet of the rest of our lives, knowing we were no longer in a position to decide what came next.

Many of my friends, fraternity brothers and fellow students either were gripped with patriotic fever and ran to enlist, or simply didn't like the anxious feeling of sitting and waiting to be called up and decided they might as well get it over with. At least they could pick their branch of service and join on their own time, although no one had any idea when exactly they might be leaving or where they were going or when or if they might be coming back.

I really wanted to finish my studies and reluctantly decided to adopt a wait-and-see stance. It made studying and attending classes difficult, not knowing if each day I would come home to find a letter telling me to drop my books and report for duty. Every day that passed without a letter from Uncle Sam put me one step closer to graduation. It was hard to concentrate with all the momentous events tugging at the world and my own life.

The days plodded along with the war casting a gloom over campus and at the same time adding urgency to the most mundane tasks. Then one day something happened that brightened the winter gray. I received a bundle of newspapers from my father, who was nice enough to send the Joliet Herald News to keep me abreast of happenings in our hometown. Sometimes there was news of Joliet Township

High School's award-winning marching band, or of some problem at one of the prisons for which Joliet is infamous. These days there were lots of stories about who was enlisting and or being drafted. Too many of my friends were putting on uniforms. I couldn't help but feel guilty at times that I was safe in my frat house and wouldn't be facing enemy bullets as soon as many of the guys I knew.

It was the February 8, 1942 edition of the *Herald News* that caught my eye. I couldn't imagine that one photo could so change my life. On the front page was a picture of a young woman holding a clock. She was looking at its face, set for two o'clock. Just below the photograph and in bold print were the words, **"Time to Move Ahead for War."** The rest of the caption read: "Miss Gertrude Pisut, 653 Henderson avenue, is not planning on staying up until 2 o'clock tomorrow morning, so she is getting ready to turn her timepiece ahead one hour tonight. The change to fast 'war time' is a national movement to conserve electricity by saving daylight."

Daylight saving time had been around as long as I could remember, but in 1942 it changed early.

I was acquainted with Miss Pisut. We had attended the same high school and both had graduated in the class of '39. I had never spoken to her and at that large school barely knew who she was, but something about her photo in the paper captivated me. Maybe she had grown from schoolgirl to woman in those few years since graduation.

Down at the bottom of that same page was a column called "Street Comment" and the question of the day was "Would you give blood to a blood bank for the army?" Among the respondents was Gertrude Pisut of 653 Henderson Avenue, who said, "I certainly would give blood to a blood bank for the soldiers, and also for the Navy. Donating blood would be something, wouldn't it? Let me know when they want it."

I hung her photo above my desk and stared at it for hours. The lovely face with hair so carefully placed, the well-pressed collar of her white blouse outlining her neck, and the neat-appearing suit coat made quite a picture. I studied every detail down to the nail polish on her hand holding the clock. "Do I dare write to her?" I asked myself over and over again.

I obsessed over the photo for days. Was it crazy for me to approach her this way? Was I being a romantic fool, or just a fool? I could hear the voice of my sister Vida in my head quoting the old cliché she said so often, "An opportunity may only knock once."

Nothing ventured, nothing gained. When I got my courage up, after thinking about that photograph and agonizing about it for over a week, I wrote to her.

March 12, 1942

Dear Gertie:

I imagine when you open this letter, you will be amazed and somewhat puzzled. I know I haven't any right to just start writing to a girl whom I don't really know except to say "hello" but I have seen you so often in the corridors at the high school, and I always wanted an introduction. Therefore, you can understand my brazen undertaking—I hope. Your picture adorns the wall to my right but the clock spoils the effect produced on the observer. Nevertheless, it is something to show the other fellows in my room since their girls aren't anything to look at. How's that for a start?

I can't think of anything more uninteresting than to discuss school with a person so close to one. Illinois is a swell place but I still think Joliet is the best. The only factor that makes this institution livable and exciting is the ever-persistent activities. There is always something going on and if you miss any event, one feels as if he has lost a million dollars. Well, maybe, it isn't that bad but you know what I mean.

Speaking about you, how is work? Tiresome I imagine, but I suppose you provide enough excitement for the students when you walk the halls. I was wondering if the new superintendent was as ornery as Jordan. If he is, God bless the school.

Well, it is time to start studying again. I think I am just wearing myself to a frazzle. Anyhow, that's what I tell my Dad, but of course, a little white lie never hurt anyone. I'll close and hope to hear from you soon."

Yours,

Dick Zalar

I included a P.S. with my address and then a P.P.S. which said:

I hope you aren't married as yet. Most of the girls in Joliet are, at the present, so I'm just curious.

I don't recall how I was aware of it, but I knew Trude was working in the superintendent's office at the high school, as secretary to Mr. Dale Dudley Coyle, who oversaw the teachers of the "Commercial" Department—which meant the business classes. Bob Gaspich, with whom I had been friends since childhood, was then a student at Joliet Junior College, which was part of the high school complex. I had written to him after I had received the paper and told him of the photograph and how it impressed me. I asked Bob to go to her office on some pretext and, without making it obvious, look her over for me. His reply was swift and sure: "If you don't date her, I will."

I spent nervous days awaiting her reply. I really knew nothing about her, including if she had a boyfriend or fiancée. Or if she would think I was crazy or weird for writing to her out of the blue like that. After a week passed, my hopes dimmed. It didn't take that long for a letter to get to Joliet and one to come back to Champaign.

Ten days later, I received a letter postmarked from Joliet and with her name in the top left hand corner of the envelope. I literally tore the envelope open.

March 22, 1942

Dear Dick:

Yes, you're wrong in thinking that I forgot about answering your letter. I thought every evening about writing since receiving your very complimentary letter, but working evenings at the dear old school handicapped me a great deal.

I was amazed and thrilled about receiving your letter. Seeing the post-mark, "Champaign, Illinois" certainly aroused my curiosity as to the sender. When seeing your name it wasn't a strange one. So, I feel as if I know you. I haven't met you formally but my sister Ag has through Sue.

About the picture in the Herald News I feel highly honored in having it exposed to view in your room. I never thought it would travel that far. It rated a bouquet of lovely flowers from my "boss" at school. Was quite thrilled about it.

Illinois must be a grand place. (Glad you think Joliet can't be beat.) I always envied anyone who had a chance to go away to school. Do most students attend school for social reasons? That is my impression.

I don't suppose it is your reason, or is it? Incidentally, in what are you majoring?

About work, it's dull monotonous, uninteresting, etc., about 3/4ths of the time. The other 1/4th (which includes lunch, Saturday mornings, coming & leaving) is more enjoyable. Many times I feel like leaving. I never did like to work in one place more than a year, even though your salary increases each year. Prefer working in places where one comes in contact with older people instead of high school students, for several reasons.

Dr. Wheat is well-liked by all I know. Had occasion to work for him for 2 days (when Miss Hamilton, his secretary, was in the hospital). Enjoyed working very much. Found he is considerate, very friendly, and has a sense of humor.

No, I am not married which is quite advantageous at a time like this, (being able to answer letters received from handsome college men). I think it is foolish for anyone to contemplate marriage at a time like this, with men enlisting and being drafted by the hundreds. What are your chances of completing your education, and not entering military service?

Guess I'll have to bid you adieu. Enjoyed spending this time in writing you. (gee it rhymes). Hope to hear from you very soon. Wish we had more in common; would make writing more interesting.

Yours,

Trude

P.S. "How do you like my new nickname? The kids thought Gert and Gertie too common so they decided to christen me, Trude.

The Sue she mentioned was the housekeeper for my family in Joliet while I was in high school. Sue lived on the East Side of Joliet, near Trude. We both referred to the university as "Illinois" as was common. Although she spelled it "Trude," taking the second half of her name, I later learned it was pronounced like the more traditionally-spelled "Trudy" which is how many people spelled it even when referring to Trude.

I have often marveled at fate. How seeing that one photo could set my life off in a direction I had never dreamed. Many times over the years I would think back to this wonderful scene in her and my life and puzzle at the irony of Pearl Harbor and that date which will live in infamy of December 7, 1941. World War II started for the US with that horrific attack on a place that was not very well known to many of us. If it hadn't, then "War Time" would not have been necessary, Trude would never have had her photograph in the Herald News where I could see it and I would never have written to her. I do wonder what my life would have been like without Gertrude Catherine Pisut. If I had never seen the photograph of her, I can't imagine how our paths would otherwise have crossed.

Many years later, after Trude was too ill to tell me of the things she had stored away, I discovered a most interesting box. We had moved seven times over the course of our marriage, and I guess Trude always took charge of this special box.

If this box was to be given any special care or to be saved for a reason, Trude had never told me or if she had, I hadn't paid attention. I know she didn't tell me what was inside or I would definitely have taken note. Had I known what was in this box, I would have opened it for a look over the years and not waited until we had moved to California and I had very reluctantly put Trude into a nursing home. The surprise wouldn't have been as great as it was when I cut open those three wide brown tape straps.

I carefully removed the tape and opened the box. I found it filled with an array of papers, cards, certificates, prayer cards and letters all neatly arranged in Trude's way. I just stood there for a moment, stunned by the treasure I had uncovered. But most striking were the bundles of letters.

Eight stacks of letters, forty or so in each packet neatly tied with a white ribbon and addressed to Miss Gertrude Pisut or Mr. Richard W. Zalar and some to Pfc. Richard W. Zalar. Some were sent to 653 Henderson Avenue, Joliet, Illinois, some to SAE fraternity house, 211 E. Daniels Street, Champaign, Illinois, others to 841 Michigan

Avenue, Chicago, Illinois, and 626 S. Ashland Avenue, Chicago, Illinois. All of the addresses we had each used during the years of our courtship. She had collected and saved every one. I have no idea where I had kept those she sent to me, and when I gave the whole lot to her. They were our letters, our love letters, which she had kept hidden away from prying eyes—mine included. And now they were there before me again. There was a total of 347, with the first dated March 12, 1942 and the last written at 9:37 p.m., and dated, September 10, 1944, six days before our marriage.

She saved everything. I found her confirmation certificate from May 31, 1934 stating that Trude, age 13, was confirmed at Sts. Cyril and Methodius Church in Joliet.

I also found a letter of recommendation written to the Dean by the Commercial Office manager at Joliet Township High School, Dale Dudley Coyle. It led to her being hired as a secretary in his department when she was nineteen years old. It read:

> *Dear Dean Haggard:*
>
> *Miss Pisut was one of six outstanding senior girls in the class of 1939, selected to work in the office in the closing weeks of the school year.*
>
> *Miss Pisut was one of two members in this group who stood as superior. In all of this service, she showed unusual ability and impressed me as possessing unusual qualifications for success as stenographer or secretary. Her typing is clean and even; she takes dictation accurately and conducts herself with excellent poise for her years. I believe her switchboard and information desk personality to be pleasing and suitable. Miss Clow is vigorous in her recommendation.*
>
> *Miss Lane speaks highly of typing done for the salary schedule committee; likewise, Mr. Deam for typing done for his latest publication. Mr. Tom Lauer was pleased with her work in his office during his secretary's vacation. Mr. Gesell, manager of Woolworth's store where Miss Pisut is now employed speaks well of her. Therefore, I wish to recommend appointment of Miss Pisut to begin work in my office Monday October 7th.*

I also found her old yearbooks. I was surprised to see that Gertrude Pisut was standing in front of me in an honor society photo taken our senior year. If I had known her in high school and somehow had found the courage to ask her out, what were the chances our romance would have lasted through the semester, let alone beyond high school? High school dating is so transient and temporary, if I had met her somehow then I might have killed whatever hope there was to make it last. So fate had also played a hand in keeping us apart until the time was right. And strangely, while the rest of the world was going to hell, the time was right for us.

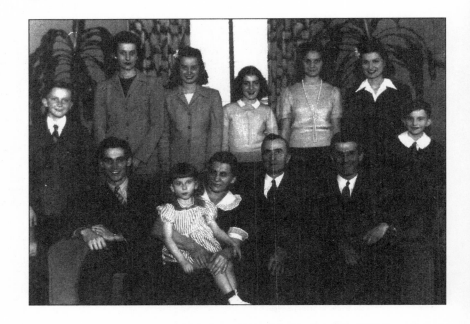

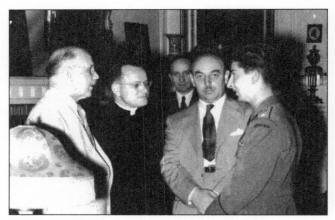

The Pisut family (top); Trude is standing back right.

My Poppa (far left), meeting with King Peter of
Yugoslavia (far right) and other Slovenian leaders.

Growing Up in Joliet

That box of memorabilia gave me a great deal of insight into Trude's early life and brought back many memories of my own childhood. We were both raised in Joliet, Illinois; she was born there in February of 1921, and I was born there a year and half later in July of '22.

Joliet was a blue-collar-worker city about 40 miles south of Chicago and was known for a few things while I was growing up: the two prisons; the school band which traveled widely representing the city; and a spectacular movie house, the Rialto, which was out of place in this town of 33,000 people. And Joliet was known for its heavy industry: the Elgin, Joliet and Eastern Railroad (known locally as the E, J & E), a US Steel plant, the Ruberoid Company, and a brick-yard employed many of the blue-collar workers who lived east of the Des Plaines River. The other big employer in town was Gerlach-Barklow, which made greeting cards. Today Chicago's suburbs have sprawled out to engulf Joliet, but back then it was an island of industry in a sea of farmland.

The Des Plaines River, like many that ran through industrial cities in those days before environmental protection, was seriously polluted. The city's sewers also emptied into the river and it often smelled like an open cesspool. In Joliet, we substituted "river" for tracks in the old expression "from the wrong side of the tracks," although train tracks abounded in East Joliet and the workers lived among them.

I grew up on the west side of Joliet, which was more residential and considered more desirable because the houses were not surrounded by mills and rail and brick yards. I didn't know Trude when I lived in Joliet and generally had little contact with the people who lived on the blue-collar side of town. Not that my family was wealthy or snobs. Far from it, but my Poppa, Joseph Zalar, did work in the white-collar world and had connections, both political and social because of his job.

He was head of the KSKJ, which in Slovenian stood for The Grand Carniolian Slovenian Catholic Union of the United States of America, or at least was part of that long title. What that meant was that in a town that was heavily populated by Eastern Europeans this Union provided support services and social activities for immigrants from that part of the world and their descendants. In those days, before labor unions and company benefits, the mills and mines would often not even pay to bury someone killed on the job or take care of the worker or his family if he was injured, so one of the primary functions was to provide insurance for families who were hit by such a tragedy. They also provided a sort of social club and cultural anchor for immigrants in the new and sometimes unfamiliar world.

In 1899, at the age of 20, Poppa came from the area of the Austro-Hungarian Empire which became Yugoslavia after World War I, and now is the nation of Slovenia. He went to work in the coal mines of Forest City, Pennsylvania, which hired many Eastern Europeans to fill the dangerous shafts. It was in these rugged surroundings that he met and married my mother, and shortly thereafter they moved to Joliet.

He started working for the KSKJ and from 1908 until his death in 1959 ran the organization as its highest salaried official. The group had been founded in 1894 and reached its peak in about 1939 with 36,000 members in 21 states and total assets in excess of $4.4 million. The group still exists in Joliet and elsewhere, but on a much smaller scale. Poppa went regularly to meet with other Slovene leaders in Cleveland, Pittsburgh, Eveleth, Minnesota, Sheboygan, Wisconsin and Pueblo, Colorado, and other cities that were prominent in KSKJ politics, and he often traveled the short distance to Chicago to meet with the groups there. Over the next 50 years, his salary grew so that in the 1940s he was making $200 a month, and when he died in 1959, he was earning $10,000 annually. True, it wasn't a lot of money on which to support a family of six kids, but it was enough to provide a good home and he loved his work and that was important to Poppa. His hard work providing much-needed services earned him the respect of many both in the Slovenian community and the rest of Joliet.

Poppa's prominent position led him to get involved in Republican politics and eventually he was elected to the Will County Board of Supervisors. Joliet is the seat of Will County. At one point he was president of the Will County Forest Preserve Board and the "Zalar Woods" preserve on the east side of Joliet was named for him in recognition of his service. He even attended the inauguration of Dwight Eisenhower in Washington, D.C., in January 1953. My father's position as a community leader in the U.S. once got him invited to meet the king of Yugoslavia. My brother Joe had also briefly dabbled in local politics but failed in his bid for supervisor. The Zalar name still raises a smile and a nod of the head in some circles in Joliet.

Zalar is pronounced to rhyme with "dollar," which some of my friends have shortened it to "Zal" to rhyme with "doll," or some have clipped it even further: Russ Stevens calls me simply "Z," and years later my son-in-law, Ron Wesoloski, made it "Dr. Z."

In 1899, when she was 13, my mother came from the section of Europe that would later be Slovenia. Her sudden death in 1925 at the age of 40 was a loss I couldn't really comprehend since I was only three at the time. As was usual in that era, the mother held the family together, but somehow my father and my siblings were able to keep us going. For a couple of years when things got to be a bit too much, I was put in an orphanage, but I moved back home when it was arranged for me to start school a year early, at age 5, since there wasn't anyone at home to look after me.

We weren't wealthy but my father managed to send my oldest brother, Joseph, Jr., to medical school, my other brother, Hubert, to law school, my oldest sister to college in Indiana, and me to the University of Illinois for my third year of college, and on to medical school, although the Army picked up the tab for the last 24 months of that. Our education and future had to be assured as well as could be with the resources at hand. His courage and stick-to-it-iveness made it so. When he was growing up, his father provided a higher level of schooling for him in the gymnasium format of learning in the town Ljubljana, 6 kilometers from his own small town in Slovenia. My siblings and I were expected to do well in school and take advantage of the much more advanced opportunities life had given us in the US. Poppa would have it no other way at our home on Nicholson Street in Joliet. Like many of that generation and background, he played the role of the autocrat in the family. He may not have been the warmest man, but he provided a solid foundation on which his children could build their lives.

As the youngest of six children I was somewhat doted upon and a little spoiled by my big sisters, who tried to make up for the nurturing I had missed due to my mother's absence. Marion, the oldest, married a man named Fran Curry, who with his many connections, did me a few favors over the years. Marion suffered from Alzheimer's disease before finally dying of it at age 87.

My sister Vida was the athlete of the family, and was also talented in the song and dance department. She dressed me correctly—or at least in ways she thought were correct—when I went out on dates with Trude and she always let me use her car for my courting as well. She lived with another nurse-friend in Cleveland. She moved back to Joliet and died there at the age of 75.

Dolores, the youngest girl, was an entrepreneur. She eloped to Cleveland at age 21. Her husband came from a well-to-do family of Slovenian heritage, which I'm sure made my Poppa happy. She was a terrific person, and could she cook! Must have learned from my Momma. She died at age 81 of cancer but she was beginning to show signs of Alzheimer's, also.

Joseph, my oldest brother, was a physician and enjoyed a very good life: he was a sports enthusiast and a card player, and was always eager to keep up with his education in medicine. One of his proudest moments was bowling a 300 game in league competition. He married, had four children of his own and lived to be 80. He was well-known in Joliet; to this day his old patients will mention him to me.

My brother Hubert was a lawyer who also loved to play cards and was an expert bridge player. He died in Florida of pneumonia and a stomach hemorrhage at age 67 without showing any signs of the dread disease that seemed to plague our family.

My father was a meticulous man who always dressed very well. He lived as a widower for 34 years and, although he had a girlfriend for years, he never remarried.

Trude was from the East Side of Joliet. Some of my friends, and even one of my sisters thought that alone disqualified her. I even heard some people say they didn't think Trude would be able to fit in a white-collar world and act like a lady. Such were the petty prejudices of the time.

Her parents were of Czechoslovak origin and came to this country at early ages. Matthias, "Matt," her father, came to Joliet when he was 14, and worked in a mill and then a dry-cleaning plant until he decided to go to school to become a funeral director. At first he associated with another establishment, but after a few years of experience, he started his own business. The part of Joliet where the family lived had a large population of Czechs and Slovaks, and they wanted to be buried with the customs of their native land and Catholic religion. He provided that service so well that the business ran for 50 years, later being operated by his son and grandson. It's still partially active today. Pisut pronounced in the Czech comes out as almost "pea-shoot."

Matt Pisut soon became well-known in Joliet and was often called upon to assist Czech and Slovak immigrants who weren't fluent in English or needed help with immigration papers or other personal matters. Much more than an undertaker, he was an advisor to many families in times of need that did not include the loss of a loved one. How he found time for all of this with his own large household to care for amazed me.

In the Pisut home there were 10 children, and Trude was third-oldest. The two-story frame home could not have been more than 1500 square feet, and it was very simply decorated with wedding photographs of her parents on the wall of the living room, along with a few religious icons. To say the least, there were crowded conditions, but somehow they got along and matured into a close-knit group of sisters and brothers. Trude was the most accomplished of them all, with her sister Mary Helen coming in a close second.

Anna Mae, "Ann," was an avid Cubs fan and a marvelous hostess—just a fun person. Mary Helen developed an amazing talent for sports—golf, bowling, and trap-shooting, in which she gained a reputation as a national champion. Theresa had a winning smile and a special charm about her.

Of the four sons, Steve followed in his father's footsteps, taking over the funeral home when Matt retired, but he did not last long at this post dying shortly after taking over at the age of 52. Steve's son took over the business. Matt, Jr. distinguished himself in the Army Air Corps during World War II, at one time providing ground support on the island of Tinian for the Enola Gay, which dropped the first atomic bomb. Clement spent 29 years as an air-traffic controller for the Strategic Air Command, and Emory also went into aviation, retiring after a long career in the airline business.

One of the biggest problems in that house on Henderson Avenue next to the funeral home was insufficient bedroom space. Five growing girls crammed into one of the three bedrooms in the home faced a daily challenge in just getting dressed without falling over each other. It also must have been a lot of fun with only a single bathroom—one toilet and one tub for 12 people. Fortunately, the mother, Helen, made everything work, and in our religious jargon anyone who did the impossible was said to be a "saint." Surely, Trude's Mom fit that description to keep things happy in such tight quarters.

To add to Helen's burden and test her saintly attributes, the youngest daughter, Barbara, was born mentally disabled and couldn't do anything for herself except rock back and forth incessantly. She was never capable of speaking, other than making unintelligible sounds. (When Barb was about 5 or so, I had arranged for the family to bring her to the medical school in Chicago and a specialist found she was born without a vital part of brain and there would be no treatment even now, and certainly wasn't back then.) There was a 16-year age difference between Trude and Barbara. Their mother cared for Barbara 24-hours a day and never complained once. Barbara lived to be 53 years of age and they would never have heard of putting Barbara in a home or care facility. The family took care of her for all of those years.

The oldest sister, Agatha, was sort of a second mother to the bunch and provided the nurturing in their mother's absence. Ag had always dressed very well, and because she spent so much time at home, became quite the collector of old movies.

When their father died, he wasn't terribly well off, but most of the money he did have, he left for the care of Barbara. Ag never married, so after Helen's death the responsibility for Barbara's care fell to her, and she tended house for her father until he and Barbara died, then followed them not many years after.

Home was surely not the quietest place to study for school but Trude did what she had to do. Among the things I found in that special box was a copy of her transcript that showed excellent scores and a ranking that I am sure must have made her parents proud. Trude never told me how well she had done in school. She didn't need to brag about such things.

She had graduated ranked 38 in a class of 570 students with a 4.3 grade-point average and was the sixth highest-ranking girl who graduated in the class of 1939. I'm a little embarrassed to say that neither my class standing nor my GPA came close to hers. I also noticed the words "cited for honesty" at the top of her transcript along with the date 11-4-36. That entry on her record impressed me very much because it said so many things about her. Even at age 15, she had good character.

Because of Mr. Pisut's work as a funeral director, the family developed a close relationship with their church, and even though she was only 9 years old, Trude then still called "Gertie," got a Saturday job scrubbing the floor in the sacristy, learning to work hard even at a young age.

As part of the graduation ritual from high school, autograph albums were popular with the girls. All of the trite little gems that were used at that time were written to Trude by her friends:

California raises oranges, Florida raises grapefruit, but only Illinois can
raise a peach like you.

Remember well and bear in mind,
a good true friend is hard to find
and when you find one just and true,
change not the old one for the new.

In your golden chain of friendship, please consider me one of its fondest
links.

God bless! the man who takes your hand,
and to the altar leads you.
But damn the man who takes your hand
and then forgets to feed you.

Like most girls of the day, Trude tried cigarette smoking. She and her friend Viv would try to shoo the smoke out the window before her mother came in the room, but Mrs. Pisut was too sharp a woman not to have known what was going on, I'm sure.

Money was always very tight for her large family, and opportunities for her to travel or do many exciting things were limited. For Trude, a thing like saving up for a charm for her bracelet was a big deal, and she was proud of the charm bracelet she put together over the years.

Trude's first job after she graduated from high school in 1939 was at Woolworth's 5&10 in downtown Joliet with pay of 37 cents an hour. She worked eight hours a day, six days a week, which was common then, but she was working and bringing home a paycheck to help the family, which was no small accomplishment during the Depression, so she couldn't complain, and didn't. One day, as she was window shopping at the stores along Chicago Street in downtown Joliet, a "Guess the number of beans in the jar" contest caught her eye. She guessed 670 and won a Helbros wristwatch that still keeps good time.

The Great Depression hit Joliet very hard, since much of the work was in heavy industries and much of the labor force was made up of recent immigrants with minimal education who had little chance of getting work elsewhere. Bread and soup lines were quite long at the city's available shelters. I lost my $25 life savings in a bank closure and at 9 years old was devastated. Every day I could see how much worse it was for people who were living on the streets because they had really lost everything. Any work that paid any money was acceptable in those dark days. Another strange irony of World War II is that had it not come along, it's hard to picture how Joliet would have gotten out of the Depression.

My first two years of study after high school were in my hometown at a respected institution, Joliet Junior College (JJC). Word was that it was the oldest community college in the country, having been founded in 1901. When I was there, it had a student body of about 250 and it was still attached to Joliet Township High School (JTHS) which Trude and I had attended.

One of the exciting events taking place in the town was "Bank Night" held at the Rialto Theater. Most anyone in town could win, since filling out an entry blank was all that was required. It was added to hundreds of others in a large metal barrel that was spun and the winner drawn on a Saturday at 9 p.m. The winner had to be present to claim the prize. Everyone dreamed of taking home the several hundreds of dollars to offset some of the financial setbacks we all suffered during the 1930's.

One dateless evening while I was still in school at JJC, my friend Jim Faulkner and I were bored and had no interest in the movie then playing at the Rialto, so we decided to cruise the downtown streets looking for something in the female line, as we liked to say. We passed the theater a number of times as we drove up and down Chicago Street in Jim's father's maroon Ford convertible—a great cruising vehicle if ever there was one—and that was the evening my name was drawn by the theater manager for Bank Night. The prize was $700. It would have covered most of my expense at school the next year when I went south to the University of Illinois. I could never live that disappointment down since almost every Saturday I went to one of the theaters to see a movie, but not that one night that it mattered. And in a town as small as Joliet was, there were lots of people who knew me and who had heard my name called and knew what I had missed.

That fall I moved to Champaign to begin my college career in earnest as a junior in pre-med. Jim Faulkner had already completed two years at JJC and a year at U of I, Champaign-Urbana. He suggested that it was better to join a fraternity than to try to live in a rooming house or a dormitory for many reasons. It cost $54 a month, which provided me not only with room and board, but a social life as well. I opted for the frat life, and my Poppa supported it. I joined one of the oldest Greek houses in the country, Sigma Alpha Epsilon (SAE) which had its origins in Alabama in the late 1800s.

My father visited me for special events at the school, like Parents' Day. He had never had a chance to experience college life and enjoyed getting a taste of it. I purchased tickets to see the football game that was part of the day's activities. He got caught up in the spirit of the crowd and had a good time, although, like most Catholics in those days and especially those from that part of the country, he was really a Notre Dame fan. (Many years later, the movie "Rudy" would capture Joliet's obsession with the Fighting Irish rather nicely.) After the game, I took him on a tour to see what living at the fraternity house was all about. Poppa took it all in with a smile. Following a nice meal, he headed back to Joliet, two hours north.

After he left, one of my better friends at the house said to me, "Your Dad was quite a man. I liked that curled moustache and his dress code. He must be a big executive back home. And how many of those cigars does he smoke a day?"

I said, "Ten. And they're Dutch Masters!" My father always projected an air of dapper prosperity wherever he went and smoked the most popular cigar of the day.

I appreciated that he wanted to share a bit of my college life, and I enjoyed being able to show him a good time on campus. I was also grateful for his financial support and the moral support that thoughtful little gestures like the newspapers from home provided. And of course, I'll always be thankful for that one paper in particular that changed my life.

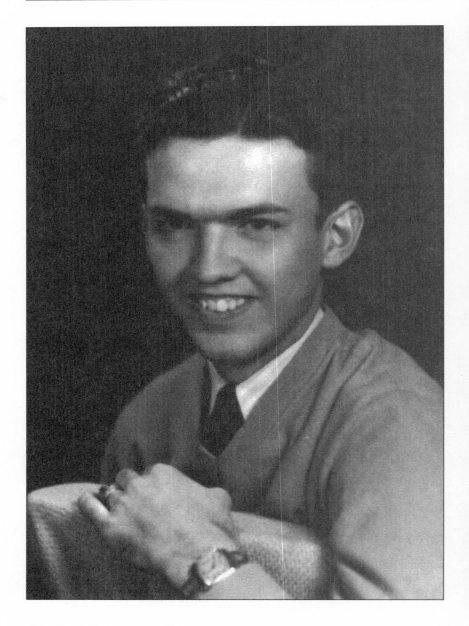

Me, Dick Zalar, as a college man.

The Elusive First Date

In my second letter, I told Trude I would be home for Easter, which was the first Sunday of April in 1942. I told her I would phone her when I got to Joliet and said so in my note:

Sigma Alpha Epsilon

211 East Daniels Street

Champaign, Illinois

Thursday, March 26th

Dear Trude:

I received your letter the other day and your immediate response was fully appreciated. I didn't think you would answer so soon, since our relationship was so limited at my first writing, but I was glad to hear from you. (You see I don't hear from home too often, if you get what I mean.)

I guess the worst subject to write on in a letter is school, but since that is my whole life down here, I think I might well discuss that as anything. Since I am in the pre-medic school, I find all the subjects mighty tough and I haven't even started into the actual work as yet. God help me! Many of my friends in the fraternity house chide me about being a "quack" because I am not too brilliant, but I just let it go at that and tell them to wait a while before making rash statements.

What do you do for excitement in Joliet? I know your work helps keep you busy, but there must be a little outside recreation for a good-looking girl. Better not overdo it or I won't have a chance to go out with you when I get home. When I do arrive in the dear old town Good Friday, I will give you a ring, and maybe we can do something over the week-end. What do you say?

You stated that I met your sister Ag thru Sue, our maid, but doggone if I can remember when or where. It probably was at the house and I can't remember names too well after only one introduction. I'll ask Sue when I see her to verify the statement.

Well, I got (swell verb from a college student) a lot of work to do, so I'll finish this masterpiece. Write soon and I'll call you.

Yours,

Dick

P.S. I like your new nickname.

I played up the sympathy saying I didn't get many letters from home. Apparently she answered my letter almost as soon as she got it, which I took as a very promising sign.

April 1

Dear Dick,

Talk about people answering correspondence promptly, I think you should be placed in that category also. I've acquired the habit since many friends have entered the service, air corps and army, no navy yet which resulted in more leisure time, and immediate replies to their letters. (patriotism??)

As to diversions in this dull city, we surprisingly find many exciting things to do. This past month, roller-skating topped the list, since dancing was prohibited during lent (religious person, you know). Being invited out for chicken and eating cheese sandwiches instead was quite amusing the other night. They didn't know we couldn't eat meat.

Guess what? Am learning to play "crap." (I think that's spelled correctly.) Received first lesson at Sprague's the other night after work. Don't think we'll receive another, kids thought it wasn't very ladylike, our learning to play that dice game.

Speaking of the new superintendent, I understand (by way of the grapevine) that the J.C. students really dislike him. He spoke to them at an assembly at which he enumerated only their poor points. Called them "disturbing elements" and inferred that they were the cause of Miss Dillman's [the librarian] death. (Please don't quote me on any of this information.)

*His speech upset the students greatly, which resulted in a 2-hr. conference
with about 7 of the Jr. Col. Boys in the superintendent's office.*

*He contemplated changing the Jr. Col. Lockers to the 2nd cross-corridor
on the 2nd floor near the shops, where they would not disturb classes, and
where Dean Yaggy could keep an eye on them.*

*Dr. Wheat's going to speak to them this noon. Perhaps this speech will
not be one-sided. Will hear about this assembly tomorrow.*

*I strongly disagree with you when you say the worst subject to write on
in a letter is school. I find it very interesting and would like to hear more
about it, especially the social phase.*

*Am looking forward to your phone call when you arrive in town. About
my overdoing it (amusement) that's impossible. Sorry to say I will not be in
town on Friday (Receiving ½ of the week's Easter vacation the school has,
beginning Friday). Going to Chicago with a friend. Will be at home
Saturday and Sunday though, eagerly awaiting your call.*

Yours,

Trude

Somehow we weren't able to coordinate our schedules over the
weekend and never met up. Our budding romance was stalled. We
just got our signals crossed and never managed to connect for reasons
that are unclear now. I wrote back to her on Easter evening, as soon
as I got back to school and the fraternity house.

Sunday Nite

Dear Trude,

*I just got in and figured I had better make up for my terrific mistake
which occurred over the weekend. I know you think that I didn't want to go
out with you, but you are very wrong in that category. I would have enjoyed
a date with you very much, but I guess it was my blundering which pre-
vented it. Please excuse it.*

*I have a very important request to make. If it is in any way possible, I
would like for you to come down to our fraternity formal, the 24th of April.
It is on a Friday and starts about 9. A friend of mine, who is a brother, is
also having his "girl" down so if you could come, I think both of you could*

*get together. Of course, she's in high school, but that wouldn't make much
difference. We also have a picnic Saturday afternoon, a radio dance
Saturday night, a formal dinner Sunday evening, and other interesting
events.*

*I sure would appreciate your acceptance, and I know that if you "beg"
Dr. Wheat for a slight leave of absence, he would permit it. Till I hear from
you, which is very soon, I hope, I remain,*

> *Yours,*
>
> *Dick*

A "radio dance" was one in which we danced to Big Band music
being played over the radio. If you didn't have the funds to hire a
band, listening to one of the popular ones of that day—Glenn Miller,
Jimmy and Tommy Dorsey, Benny Goodman, and their like—was a
good substitute, and some radio stations broadcast programs called
things like "Saturday Night Dance Party."

After my mistake of not calling her over the weekend I wasn't sure
I'd ever hear from her again. But on April 7, she wrote back to me:

> *Tuesday Noon*
>
> *Dear Dick,*
>
> *Soon is the word. Just couldn't allow another hour to tick away without
> answering your "super" letter. Excitement leaves me speechless, but here goes.*
>
> *That very important request of yours simply left me stunned. Have had
> time to recover, and think it will be a thrilling experience to attend your fra-
> ternity formal. Something out-of-the-ordinary. I ought to repeat that, but I
> won't. Would like very much to accept instantly, but as usual, regretfully I
> may say, several factors will have to be taken into consideration before doing
> so. Don't misunderstand, am not leading to a negative answer. Hope I will
> not be forced to decline your invitation.*
>
> *First of all, in black & white, how many days leave would I need?
> Saturday a.m. I hope is all. It is quite difficult to be excused on a school day,
> Friday. Might be able to arrange for Friday noon. But how does one expect
> me to be calm-and-collected Friday morning? What time Friday would you
> recommend leaving to arrive at a leisurely hour?*

Who is your fraternity brother? His girlfriend? Will have to look her up. What did you mean by the remark of her being in high school not making much difference?

Back in work tomorrow after a fine vacation. Too short, though. Will ask the "boss" about Friday & Saturday. Have my doubts, as I am an invaluable element in that institution. Hmm-m-m-m!

About the weekend (last), just erase it from your mind. Very stupid of me, really. Should have remained at home Sat. to begin with.

Don't overwork. Find time to answer very soon. In high hopes, with fingers crossed,

Yours,

Trude

P.S. Expect my answer in next reply.

Of course I was thrilled with her response and quickly wrote back to her on my SAE stationery:

Thursday, April 9

Dear Trude:

I received your letter this morning and your reply to my invitation was swell. I hope you can come down cause I know we will have a swell time.

You asked about the details. Well, here they are. The fellow from Joliet, who is a fraternity brother, is Art Lennon. He goes with "Pete" Kennedy who attends J.T.H.S. She is coming down with another friend. Pete lives at 1207 Taylor, (I guess that number is correct, anyway, she lives on Taylor St.) so if you call her and find out when and how she is coming down, I'm sure that our plans can be completed. Tell her that I asked you to attend our dance, and that I would appreciate her helping you out. I forgot to tell you that the dance starts at 9:30, Friday nite, and we have a formal dinner about 7:30. Therefore it would be necessary to get off work Friday. I sure do hope your "boss" is in a good mood so that you can come down. I'll complete the arrangements down here as to where you are to stay, etc. as soon as I hear from you.

Answer as soon as you find out what's cookin and I'll be waiting.

Yours,

Dick

The "swells" and "what's cookin" seem comically dated now, but I can still remember how giddy I was when I wrote that letter. I was going to have the best-looking date at the SAE spring formal! Then the bottom dropped out of my high. I had to write and tell her about it. Strange how important historical dates have also had significance in our lives. Lincoln was shot and the Titanic hit an iceberg on April 14.

> *April 14, 1942*
>
> *Dear Trude,*
>
> *I know this is going to be quite a shock to you, but it is unavoidable. Just yesterday, I was informed that I was selected as a candidate or delegate to the Province Convention on the same weekend that the spring weekend is to be held. I tried to get out of it, but it was impossible. If, by chance, I can be relieved of the assignment and it is an earlier date, I will inform you and maybe we can still get together. I'm awfully sorry, but that's the way it goes, I guess. This will be the only party I could have attended, since I will not be here next year. And now this happens. I guess I wasn't born with a gold spoon in my mouth. Write when you are able and I'll see you when I get home.*
>
> *Yours,*
>
> *Dick*

As fate would have it, while I was writing to her expressing my regrets with mangled metaphors, she was writing to me.

> *Tuesday, April 14, 1942*
>
> *Dear Dick,*
>
> *Finally I received Dr. Wheat's permission to have Friday off.*
>
> *He wasn't very willing, but he consented. Jeanette is going to Ames three weeks later, and two requests for leaves in a month's time were just too much for him, during our "busy" season.*
>
> *Was able to contact "Pete" this morning after two fruitless attempts. She was very pleased to hear of the invitation, and thinks you're one grand person. I think she is very sweet & considerate. Was very eager to have me come along with her & her friend. No doubt you know they're planning on leaving*

on the 10:15 (I think, or 10:00) from Kankokee Friday, arriving at about
12:00 noon. She & her friend have arranged to stay at her sister's sorority
house; and would try to make some arrangements for me. Thought it would
be ideal for all of us to be together. Course, nothing definite has been
decided yet. Completely forgot to mention to her that you offered to make
arrangements for a place for me to stay. Would be nice, though, if we could
all be together.

"Pete" doesn't know yet that I'm able to go. Received Dr. Wheat's per-
mission after seeing her. Will see her again tomorrow. She spoke of the vari-
ous events and how fun they were. Am terribly excited and impatient.

Sorry that I was unable to reply sooner. Hope I haven't kept you in fear
of my not receiving permission for Friday off, with the eventful day but a
week away.

Am "tickled pink" that thing turned out as I hoped.

Yours,

Trude

Being naive, I thought my attendance as our fraternity's represen-
tative at the meeting in Wisconsin was mandatory and since I had
been elevated recently to an "active" position in the fraternity, I
thought I couldn't refuse. I was a junior, but a "pledge" (a status more
common with lower classmen), and some of my fraternity brothers
teased me because of this. And I guess in some ways I was still a
small-town boy ripe for ribbing. I still wonder if perhaps some of the
older brothers got tired of hearing me talk about my hot date for the
formal and concocted this whole mandatory fraternity convention
thing to get me.

April 17, 1942

Dear Trude:

I received your letter the other day and I am very sorry that we couldn't
get together. Darn it, anyway! I suppose you are ready to tear your hair after
you struggled so hard to get the day off work, but I couldn't do much about
the predicament. I sure do appreciate your attempt, but I'll make it up to
you when I get home. Please don't be too angry cause I wouldn't want to

hurt your feelings. I hope you understand. I doubt very much whether or not I will be relieved of the duty of attending the convention and then I suppose, if I could be exempted from going it would be too late to do much about it. Art got a letter from Pete the other day and she thought you were swell, (of course, I do too.) And she couldn't understand how it was possible for me to get a date with you. I guess she doesn't think I am worthy of your presence. What do you think? Now?

Well, I've got to start studying. There is an exam coming up Monday in chemistry and a lot of extra work to do before the weekend is up, so I have to hit the books early this time.

Write soon and I'll see you soon and this time there will be no mix-up.

Yours,

Dick

Naturally, I thought my chances with her for any future dating would be slim to none after such a fiasco. First there were the fumbled plans over Easter, and now this. Somehow, I was able to avoid the out-of-state travel and called her to see if she might still be able to come down for the dance. But during the time consumed for the exchange of her and my letters, she had been asked to go to the annual Military Ball to be held at the high school where she worked. It was to be on the same date as the big fraternity party. Over the phone talking about her disappointment at not being able to attend my formal, she cried, so I could just imagine how upset she must have been when she first got the news.

For a girl like Trude whose life had been quite sheltered, a fraternity formal was a big deal. She had done very little traveling, so the train trip down to Champaign in and of itself would have been exciting. Since very few of her friends were able to afford the luxury of college, she did not even have their experiences to share vicariously. Going to college was not nearly as common back then, and the chance to visit a campus, stay in a sorority house and go to a frat dance, were all going to be a wonderful interruption to what she was already beginning to see as her hum-drum life of working all day at the same place she had gone to high school, then going home to her shared room in very close quarters. She was surrounded by younger people at school and her siblings at home, so this was a chance to be around people her own age and have a great time. She took it pretty hard when I burst her bubble.

After my apologetic phone call, I got a letter from her. There was a little bit of a sharp edge to her letter, and some obvious sarcasm, but at least she was still writing to me, and I took this as a very good sign that she had not dismissed me as a complete flake. It also was the first notice I received that she was a rather determined woman who was not going to let grass grow under her feet.

> *April 21*
>
> *Dear Dick,*
>
> *Well, I'm glad that's settled. Sorry I was so hasty in accepting that other date "The Military Ball" but one doesn't get anywhere thinking things over. But you definitely stated in your last letter my chances of going to the party were very slim, since you were unable to escape the assignment, and if, by a miracle, you were, it would be too late to notify me. And I do hate receiving last minute invites. I need at least 2 weeks to prepare for an occasion as special, elaborate, unusual, exciting as your fraternity weekend.*
>
> *I do hope you enjoy yourself immensely with Miss So & So, whom you are going to ask instead, as you informed me in our phone conversation this morning. I am sure she will be pleased being able to be escorted by you. I certainly do envy her. But I wasn't born with a lucky charm, either, sad to say.*
>
> *Perhaps I was misinformed, but I heard you asked a Gamma or something—something girl to your fraternity dance when you were supposed to have asked me. And I received your letter saying you were selected as a candidate to some old convention, I was certain that it was only your way of taking me out of the picture. After all, I didn't know if it was the truth or not. I should be a skeptic, but, after all, I'm only human.*
>
> *Of course your telephone call helped matters a bit, your effort to contact me as soon as possible. Sorry I wasn't able to receive it Monday night. If I had, I wouldn't have accepted the date to "The Military Ball." Monday night I had to complete an "Evening School Report." Was busy working away when Dr. Wheat walked in. He was greatly disturbed about my hav-*

ing asked for a leave of absence, and now I was not going. Worked a while longer, but felt quite uneasy working in Dr. Wheat's presence. Left at 8:30 and with Viv went for a Coke, where we met a couple of friends. Before we knew it we had accepted the date for Friday.

Upon arriving home, was quite surprised to hear of the long distance phone call. Mother and Sis called the school to tell me about it, but I did not answer the phone, fearing it was someone who wanted a message delivered to a student in the Defense Classes. Had I answered the phone, I could be seeing you Friday. It probably turned out for the best, no doubt. Your Miss So & So will probably be more entertaining and vivacious.

You don't know how disappointed I was upon receipt of your letter in which you wrote of your selection to the convention, and my not being able to attend your party. I actually cried. Wrote a nasty letter than I dared not mail. When I told Pete about it, she was stunned. I told her of my elaborate plans and my anxiety to go, which prompted her to write that _____ letter. (Can't fill any word, I only addressed it, (letter) did not read it.)

I did believe, after reading your disappointing letter, that my chances of going were hopeless. I really didn't care to go after that. Was confident that you were highly honored in being selected to attend the convention; was sure you would not regret it. Pete thought differently. Was positive you could shake it. Guess she was right, but it was too late.

Pete was quite alarmed to hear today that I wasn't going Friday. She was more concerned about my going, it seemed, than I was myself. She hated to see me miss out on all of the fun, I guess. I think she is one of the sweetest kids I know. Don't you?

Was embarrassed informing my friends and co-workers that I wasn't going to the frat. party after all. Don't think I told everyone, though. Will be able to clear up the matter the weekend of the party, when I'll be confronted with several questions, I'm sure.

About Pete's letter to Art, her perplexity of the possibility of your getting a date with me, and your remark of not being worthy of my presence. Could it be that it was meant visa versa.

Hope you do have a lovely time this weekend. Would like very much to

hear about the affair. If you do have time, please write. Next or 2nd best is
better than nothing, I've been told.

Glad you are able to attend the spring party, since it is going to be your
one & only due to the fact that you will not be at Illinois next year.

Have fun. Twas a swell dream for me while it lasted.

Yours,

Trude

P.S. Can't wait to hear about the weekend. Will have to see Pete about it
too next Monday. It's happened twice. Hope there won't be a 3rd.

Long-distance phone calls were expensive then and just receiving
one was an event, especially to someone who could not afford them.
These days when two people are apart they think nothing of picking
up the phone. Such extravagance was unheard of then—long distance phone calls were reserved for the most important business and
kept short.

After being made to feel properly chastised and guilty, I went to
our party just to be going and dated one of the sorority girls I knew.
It was a nice affair as I told Trude in my next letter, but I was not feeling well and wasn't able to enjoy many of the events that took place.
Maybe Trude's hurt feelings gave me sympathy pain, and I didn't
want to enjoy myself. I wrote to her about it:

April 26, 1942

Dear Trude:

By the time you receive this letter, I imagine Pete will have conveyed the
weekend's festivities to you. If I were you, I would believe only half of what
I see, and nothing of what you hear.

I attended the dance, picnic and dinner, and it was swell. I didn't enjoy
it very much though because I got sick Thursday night and didn't attend
school Friday a.m. I felt lousy most of the day Friday and the pain in my
stomach still remains. I guess I proved myself to be quite a bore to my date,
she being a Gamma Phi, and I tried to keep myself from going asleep more
than once. I saw Pete and Jackie, and they sure didn't show a very friendly
attitude, but that's no skin off my nose. They're nice kids, but just kids. Pete

insists on giving advice to everyone, but she should remember the way she gives the boys back home the run-around and also my brother, Art. She ought to practice what she preaches.

I think possibly I should discuss something more interesting or else more pleasant to both of us. Your letter, I received, was very interesting and I was surprised at the length. I thought that was a novel when I first opened it, but I was glad it was so long since I hardly ever get such lengthy and enlightening letters. I hope I get some more on that order, but soon.

I think I might be home in a couple of weeks and I hope that the 3rd time is the charm. This friendship, or should I call it enmity now, has been the craziest ever. I've never met you, except by telephone conversation and letters and that doesn't do you justice I know. I'll make sure I see you next time, that is if you want me to.

If I interpreted your statement "as to being next or 2nd" correctly, I don't consider it in the same way. But I suppose if I tried to relate my feelings you would think I was giving you a line or something. After all, Pete told you about me and not to take my statements too seriously, didn't she, or hasn't she come to that stage of my life yet.

Well, I have to hit the books since my average had depleted in the past weeks, so I'll close and expect to hear from you soon.

Always,

Dick

P.S. Tell Pete to go to hell!

2 P.S. Included in the letter is an invitation which I had addressed in anticipation of your acceptance last Monday nite.

After this exchange of letters, and our obvious clash of words, including our difference of opinion over "Pete," I was not sure we would ever get together. At times this correspondence reminded me of the James Stewart-Margaret Sullavan movie "The Shop around the Corner," with its on-again, off-again romance by letter. But I figured I owed it to myself to take a chance at redeeming myself with Miss Pisut. After enough time had elapsed to let the smoke clear, I tried again, and wrote to her full of flattery and compliments:

May 1, 1942

Dear Trude:

I just finished pitching horseshoes and since it was too dark (9:30) to continue, I decided that the best thing was to write to the nicest girl I know. I suppose you'll consider that statement as part of my college line but it's the truth. I don't think I've ever met, in an indirect way, a girl who was of your caliber and in my estimation, that is darn high. I could kick myself for not having you attend our spring party, but as you said, I guess it was better, since absence makes the heart grow fonder.

Nothing of importance has occurred of late. School is still tough and my grades are terrible. I had a 4.1 last semester but I will be fortunate to hit a 3. this time. Of course, the latter may be due to the fact that I haven't been studying very much in recent weeks, but it's pretty difficult to do when it's so nice outside. During the day I play golf and at night, I go to the show or sit around and "shoot the bull" with the other fellows. I don't go out very much, in fact, I don't intend to because not many of the sorority girls are of my taste and I guess the feeling is the same in their estimation. But it doesn't bother me very much, since they are a bunch of gold-diggers and all have home town loves. (I guess I'm in the same boat. Right?)

Tomorrow we are participating in a big track meet. The winners receive points which are added to their Intramural standing and we need every one we can attain. At the present, in the all-University race we are 2nd and with only 3 weeks left, it appears that we will be unable to catch the leaders. The winner receives a large, beautiful trophy and it adds prestige to the fraternity house possessing it. Say a prayer for us, will you?

I don't know how to go about asking this question, but I'll be blunt and to the point. Would it be possible for you to attend our senior prom on May 25th? Bob Chester's Orchestra is playing and I know we could have a good time together. Please try to make it and we could go home together Tuesday a.m. I'll be out of school the 22nd, and will stay down here if you can make the date.

Well, I guess I'll hit the hay. Don't forget to write soon and I enjoy the 5 page letters.

Always,

Dick

P.S. Don't overstrain yourself in tennis cause I wouldn't want you to be
indisposed when I get home.

I could only hope she would give me one more chance and still
want to come down for that taste of college life I had promised her.
Her next letter came in a week.

Tuesday, May 5

Dear Dick,

Thank you for the very complimentary remarks. Didn't impress me as being
a part of your college line. The "line-ing-est" man I know is Mr. Coyle (boss)
and I put up with it every day. I can hang the wash on it. It's incomparable.

About the Senior Prom on the 25th. Whose idea was it to pick on a
Monday? When I informed Dale Dudley (Coyle) of the wonderful news, he
asked me to write requesting the date to be changed from Monday to
Saturday. Would be much more convenient for him & me and everyone else
in the office. (cute kid) Seriously, he is as anxious for me to have the 2 days
off as I myself am. (It would necessitate me receiving Monday and part of
Tuesday off. Right?) Told him how eager I am about going. Didn't know
whether it was wiser for him or me to see Dr. Wheat about receiving permis-
sion for the 2-days leave. Is going to sleep on it this evening.

I dread seeing Dr. Wheat. Am sure he will question me about the last
request. Why didn't I go? What happened? Friend? Bla-bla-bla. Your work?
When? Bla-bla. His wife's name is Gertrude. Always brings her into our
conversations. She and his children are in town, living in Oneida St. You
should meet her. Boy is she an odd specimen! (Me catty? No) They both were
at the Junior-Senior Prom last Friday.

Back to the subject in question. Monday and Tuesday are the last school
days of this semester, therefore are very busy days. Tuesday noon is the day
of the faculty picnic, office people attending the affair to be excused Tuesday
noon. This might help matters some. Here's hoping.

What train would you recommend my taking Monday? Time of arrival
in Joliet, Tuesday? Would really like to see the points of interest in Illinois.
Wouldn't it be swell if the prom were Sat. night? Would occupy 2 "free"
days, Sat. & Sun., instead of letting them go to waste and inconveniencing

everyone Mon. & Tues. Can't please everyone, though.

Sorry to hear of your gold-digging girl troubles. Don't believe them, though, about your home-town love, I'll have to give that statement deep thought.

Said a few prayers for you fellows participating in Intramurals. Now am confident that you will receive 1st place and the trophy. Thank you? You're welcome.

Brr-rr-rr. It's winter in the dear old city this week. It had better warm up a bit soon so that we can resume our tennis. Needn't worry about my overdoing it. Play a slow game and have a stooge to chase our balls.

Dick Jurgens is entertaining at the Rialto tomorrow. Hope we aren't disappointed.

What other occurrences in Joliet of interest? Oh yes, the Junior College Spring Formal May 15. Don't you wish you were in town to attend it?

Glad you enjoy the 5-page letters. There's a surprise in store for you in the next one, as to length. Until then,

Yours,

Trude

P.S. Why does it take 4 days for your letters to reach me? I observed your last one was dated May 1, and I received it May 4. I find it quite disturbing as I enjoy receiving them, and look forward to replying.

I was gratified by her P.S.—she liked getting my letters! That she would even consider letting me consider her my "home-town love" after my brazen attempt to slip that in there, was also very encouraging.

Of course, one of the big problems for Trude was time off from work, and if she solved that one, she had to find a way to get to Champaign, 110 miles away. Since the war was in progress travel was restricted. Gas and rubber were rationed for the few lucky enough to own cars and priority on the trains and buses was given to servicemen. Holding the dance on a Monday evening was no problem for me and the other students who would be attending since the semester would be over then. I had no idea then or now as to why they held it on such an odd night instead of a weekend night. I was beginning to wonder if she was going to be able to get the days off, or even wanted to see me, so I wrote to her:

May 18, 1942

8 p.m.

Dear Trude,

I have been waiting for a letter the past week and I came to conclusion that you are not coming down. You aren't angry at me, are you, for not agreeing with your desire to skip work? I hope not. Don't think that I have another date or something like that, cause I haven't even given it the slightest consideration. If you could make it, I would love to have you attend with me and nobody else could supplant you!

Well, we lost the Intramural race, we were defeated by 24 points and the fellows are quite glum. Boy we would have liked to win that big trophy. It sure stunned us to lose. Next year will be different, I know.

School is drawing to a close and I am not too sorry. I have had enough of it and a vacation will be well appreciated. During the next week, I will cram and cram, since the exams will cover part of the last 6 weeks work and another part, the previous 12 weeks of information. I hope I hit 'em.

Well, I'll see you soon. I'll call you as soon as I get in. Be good and write soon.

Love,

Dick

P.S. Please forgive the usage of soon, but my mind is blank at the present.

But at the same time she was writing to me and once again she was eager to come. She had gotten her hopes up for the last trip and now wanted to make them real.

Monday May 18

(10:00 p.m.)

Dear Dick,

I'm very sorry for being so neglectful. No I am not angry with you for reprimanding me for trying to skip work. How can I be?

Since last Monday I have been very busy trying to make arrangements for transportation to & from Champaign at hours agreeable to Dr. Wheat. I've finally succeeded. My luck has changed. The most wonderful thing occurred Saturday morning. Garland McGowan, to whom I spoke about my invitation to the Prom, paid me a visit Saturday. She had a letter from her date, Noel Meyer, saying that he had to leave bag and baggage from Men's Hall, where he rooms at school, before Monday the 25th, resulting in his coming home the weekend before the Prom. This more than meets with Garland's approval for she simply must attend her 13–14 pd. German class Mon. to take the last exam, before the final, of the semester. One thing is certain, she will leave late Monday noon, late enough for me to go along. Isn't it marvelous that I can really come down? The super news was so startling it left me petrified.

Another thing. Garland wishes to arrive in time for her 3—4 pd. Class Tuesday morning. So-o-o, I guess I'll get back in time for work, or almost in time. Not saying in what condition. It probably won't matter greatly, for I don't or won't feel the after-effects until noon, when the faculty will be out picnicking.

Also, she has a couple of friends attending Illinois, at whose sorority house we can dress. Can't remember the sorority at present, but will inform you in next writing, also the approximate time of arrival.

The fact that I am able to attend the prom thrills me immensely. Think I'll wear my red-and- white gown. Hope you'll like it.

Was sorry to hear that you lost the Intramural race. Losing a big shiny trophy certainly is disappointing.

Naughty, naughty. Scholars should not cram. I always did when I was in school, way back when.

One thing in your letter was very confusing—the date. May 18. 8:00 p.m. Time marches on!!, at Illinois only, of course. I received your letter and read it at 5:45 p.m. Stranger than fiction! Am sure the very near dates of exams are the cause of this oversight. (Sorry, I didn't mean to be so elaborative.)

Wish you loads and tons of luck in your exams. Between crammings, please remember to write.

Yours,

Trude (10:30 p.m.)

P.S. Here's hoping you make the grade by a wide margin.

Of course, I was thrilled that things were falling into place so nicely. Then I got another wonderful letter.

Friday May 22

Dear Dick,

Good morning! Just got in from the show. (saw one of the features before) and thought I had better write to make up for my negligence last week.

I supposed you've completed all of those dreaded exams by now. I thought of you yesterday, pondering over tough questions, and said a prayer for the answers to "pop" into your head. Did any such miracle occur? I was behind it all.

Am all set to go down Monday. Am patiently awaiting the day. Very grateful, that the transportation headache has been simplified. Thanks to dear Garland and her friend, Mr. Myers. Do you know any of them? Am going to stay with Garland's friends, who are members of the Alpha Chi Delta. I hope I have that "straight." These Greek names are all Greek to me. Betty Barber is one of the girls.

Am planning on leaving at 4:00. Arriving at 6:30? Will give you a buzz on arrival.

A few of the J.C. students were injured, not seriously, in an accident at intersection of Rte. 6 & 7 en route to Chicago yesterday. One of Miss Wolfe's classes. Clipping from Spectator enclosed.

I'm coming. Keep your shirt on! Guess Ag wants to sleep. Yawn! Yawn! Goodnight! She insists, must close.

Yours,

Trude

P.S. Will see you soon, Can't wait.

Trude once again had apparently been keeping her sister Agatha, with whom she shared a bed, awake. The other bed in that room held her other three sisters, with Theresa, the youngest, sandwiched in the middle.

Without Garland's fortuitous offer, the whole affair would probably never have happened. Once again fate took a hand. Garland even arranged for Trude to be a guest at a sorority house where she would be able to dress for the dance and where she would be able to stay that night.

Trude arrived with Garland and her date, Noel Meyer, in the late afternoon after a two and a half hour drive down from Joliet. Betty Barber, who was from Joliet and a member of the Alpha Chi Delta sorority house, a very popular girls' residence on campus, had generously taken care of all the arrangements for Trude and Garland. I called the sorority house and told her how glad I was that she was here, and I could hardly wait to meet her.

I picked her up at 8:45 p.m. at the Alpha Chi House with a friend who had a car. He already had his date with him. I went to the front door of this large two-story home that was typical of those mansions where one could picture English royalty living; I felt as if I was in another world when I stepped into the foyer. Its stateliness added to the grandeur of the night.

My first glimpse of her was spellbinding, and I wanted to hold her close to me, never to let her go. Two commonly used phrases of the time came to mind: she really "sent me" and I felt like I was on "cloud nine." She was like nothing I had ever seen before—arrayed as she was in a formal evening gown of red and white and not a hair out of place. I recalled catching brief glances of her in the corridors of our high school but had never studied her in all her beauty, and certainly not dressed like this. She had just been part of the background at the school, a piece of the general picture we accepted in our walk from class to class. And for sure, the pictures in our yearbooks didn't do her justice. But now, two years later, she had blossomed into a beauty with every thing about her provocative: her hair, her eyes, her lips, her hands with her nails beautifully contoured, her figure and the plunging neckline. She looked great. I kept thinking that in less than an hour, I would be holding her in my arms moving across the dance floor. I had purchased a corsage and I couldn't wait to pin it on her gown.

I wouldn't say I was a totally naïve 19-year-old young man from a home of rather recent immigrants, but I really didn't have that much experience with girls, let alone a woman. Trude was already 21, no longer a teenager in looks or attitude. Girls tend to mature faster emotionally anyway, and Trude was certainly ahead of me on that score.

Anything I learned of the other sex was from my friends in the field across the street from my home, where we gathered in our crudely made dug-out to sneak a Wing cigarette. The sex education there was frank and crude and often, it turned out, wrong. With that as a basis for my knowledge of women, it was no wonder I was a bit clueless and immature.

The dance was a roaring success as far as I was concerned. She was the belle of the Ball and we enjoyed each other and the music, in fact the whole evening, from start to finish. Everything from jitterbugging with, "In The Mood," the popular Glenn Miller recording which had sold millions of "platters," to cheek-to-cheek dancing to those standards "At Last" or "I Know Why" made the evening magical. Those songs were just the thing to hold a girl close with the subdued lights above and the swishing of the girls' gowns as we moved across the floor. The sensation was almost impossible to describe. I didn't want the night to end. I added to the scene by wearing my formal tails, my white starched pin collar shirt and my white self-tied bow tie. It was the first time I had worn a tux—one my sister Vida was nice enough to purchase for me for the occasion. I wore the required pair of black patent-leather shoes and a boutonniere finished the look.

From the time the dance started until the last song was winding down, many of my fraternity brothers would stop and say hello, smiling with approval on this girl from Joliet. Garland was there, as was Betty Barber, whom I knew briefly from high school. Trude and I danced to almost every piece of music Bob Chester played, and though I thought I could move pretty well on the floor, she made me move more easily. There was something about holding her that made it feel like I could do anything or that my feet were not touching the floor. I was gliding on glass like Fred Astaire.

By the time we got back to the sorority house, it was two o'clock in the morning. We talked for a few moments while I got up the courage to kiss her goodnight, which, as I remember, left me wanting more. She kissed so well. All of the clichés about violins and fireworks came to mind. I told her I'd see her soon in Joliet. She was leaving without me the next morning to get to her job at a reasonable hour. I surely hated to see her leave, but I would be back also, very soon, to continue the beginnings of our love affair.

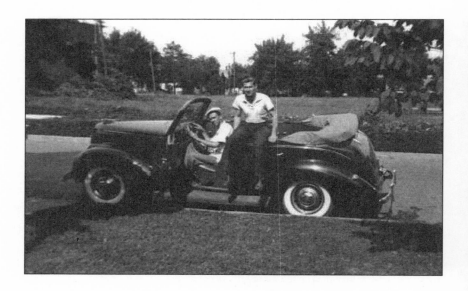

Me at the wheel and Joe
Limacher sitting on Faulkner's
convertible. (top)

Trude and her friend Viv on
their trip to Wisconsin

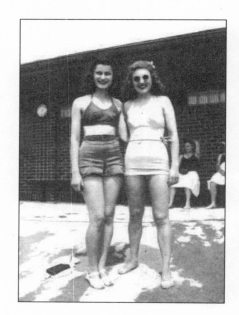

The Summer of '42

Trude and I had no reason to write once I came home the day after she did. We would be together a lot that summer, which, while lots of fun at the time, made for a gap in the wonderful string of correspondence.

That summer in Joliet with Trude was great. We regularly dated, sometimes double-dating with friends—most often Russ Stevens and his steady girl, JoAnn. Sometimes we went out with Joe Limacher and whomever he was dating at the moment, although it was rare that Joe could get a car, which was a prime consideration for double-dating. My father had a beautiful '41 Buick, my sister Vida had a Dodge, and sometimes I would borrow my brother-in-law Fran Curry's Cadillac. Russ could get his father's car more often than I could get one, which suited me fine. I liked it better when someone else drove, because then Trude and I could sit in the back and neck.

One of our dates that summer was to the amusement park, and somehow I managed to talk her into taking the parachute-drop ride even though she was terrified of heights. She screamed the whole way down and swore she'd never do it again.

With the war on, Joliet was buzzing, and the mills were working as I hadn't seen them in almost a decade. Some days the smoke hung over the city, but between doing our part for the war effort and having everyone working again, no one complained.

Some of my friends said that they didn't see much of me that summer because all of my attention was focused on Trude. I was 19 and had never really had a steady girlfriend before and was enjoying the thrill and all the perks that came with it. All of the big bands made it to Chicago, and Trude and I managed to see some of the most popular, including Benny Goodman and Glenn Miller. Sometimes we went to the Empire Room of the Palmer House to hear Griff Williams play.

With the manpower shortage that the war created, my sister Marion was having a hard time finding anyone to the work around the large house and yard she and her husband, Fran Curry, owned and they asked me if I might like a job working for them. It was basic handyman chores, painting, yard work and the like, and the pay was pretty good. But after putting in long days, often in the hot sun, I was rarely in any condition to be able to go out during the week, so Trude and I usually saved a good part of the weekend for each other. We went to the movies a lot. Before television, that was the main source of entertainment. We both loved to dance, so would go to a ballroom, preferably out of Joliet if we could—anything to break the monotony of our small town. One of our favorite trips was to the Oh Henry ballroom in Willowbrook, about 15 miles east of Joliet. We especially liked that trip when Russ drove because Trude and I had lots of backseat time.

There were parties and carnivals and other fun dates, but many evenings I sat at home, too pooped to party, just listening to the popular radio shows. Life did seem simpler when a date was often just a Coke at the local soda fountain.

We went dancing at many different places and especially enjoyed jitterbugging. Maybe my opinion is a little prejudiced, but I thought Trude and I were the best, sliding across the brilliantly polished floor under the colored lights that reflected overhead and made the scene most exciting. The credit is mainly due to her—she moved her body and those well-formed legs smoothly, gliding back and forth as I cavorted around her in a flashy fashion, our feet keeping the rhythm without missing a step. We put on quite a show. She loved the music of the era, was always up on the latest releases, and when we would go to an eating place after a movie, the jukebox at our table played incessantly. One of our favorites in the 1940s was a radio show called

"Juke Box Saturday Night," and often, we'd get up and start dancing wherever we were—soda fountain, restaurant, it wouldn't matter. I am sure the adults were shaking their heads complaining about these crazy young people.

In the '30s and the '40s going on a date often meant a movie and a snack at a drive-in or some other place that was a hangout. Dancing in Joliet was limited to the occasional church social, at which a small band would try to entertain. So when we could, we would plan a Saturday night to go somewhere special like Chicago to dance or to Aurora to see a movie and do a little night-clubbing. Because of the Depression and later the war it made just being able to get out of town a treat, and it was nice to go somewhere different at least once in a while.

We always liked to go to the Aragon ballroom, a popular dance hall in Chicago. It was built back in the 1920s and had a sister ball-room on the south side of Chicago known as the Trianon. We went there once as well. On weekends, both were crowded with young people and a few oldsters. When you entered the dancing area, the place was alive. Happy guys would take their dates by the hands and lead them from the tables where they had eaten dinner to join the swinging band and those couples already jumping to the beat on the dance floor. The big bands played at these venues, and one of our favorites was Dick Jurgens. His lead singer, Eddy Howard, was so good that when he would sing, the crowd just stopped dancing. Most everyone would stand, swaying back and forth with the music in time to Eddy's great voice. I would stand behind Trude and hug her closely with my face next to hers, wishing this could last forever but knowing it would be over in a few minutes, so I had to enjoy it while I could and savor each second. I was in heaven to have Trude's soft young body in my arms with the sweet smell of her delicate perfume mak-ing me swoon.

Morbid as it sounds, sometimes we had our dates in the Pisut Funeral Home when there were no bodies on display. In Trude's crowded house, going next door to the mortuary was often the only place to have any sort of privacy. One night, we had gone parking at Parks School, a few blocks from her home. When we finally came up for air and decided to call it a night, we were shocked to find it was almost 2 a.m. I took her to the front door of her home, and as I caressed and smooched her for the last time, she inadvertently pressed the doorbell with her back. Her father came to the door in his underwear, yelling, "What the hell is going on?" Seeing it was us, he then demanded, "What time is it?" We lied and said it was midnight. We could only hope he would go back to bed without confirming that.

Trude knew how to keep me interested and to tease. Some of the few letters I got from her that summer were when she went with her closest friend, Vivian Pironciak, to Wisconsin for a week's vacation while I wiled away the hours yearning for her return and cutting the grass at my sister's house. She wrote:

> Monday, July 6, 1942
>
> Dear Dick:
>
> Oh hum, had a very enjoyable Sunday. Just got in. It's raining cats & dogs outside this minute; in fact it has been all night.
>
> Are staying at the Ravenswood House 5 miles from the Lake Town Hotel where we were unable to get any accommodations for the evening. Has all the modern conveniences one would expect. (like ducks) Am very anxious to move into our own cottage in the morning.
>
> Spent the afternoon dancing at the Dutch Mill. Very modern. Floor perfect. Corry Lynn's orchestra furnished the music. His swingy music rates A-1. I'm sure you'd like it very much. Missed dancing with you. The gentleman I danced with practically all afternoon isn't fond of swing music. Can't jitter, the jerk.
>
> (Talking about modern conveniences, Vivian is beginning to wash for the evening. We have a basin and pitcher of water. No bathroom, running water or anything. Nuts!!)
>
> Ate at the Snack this evening. Very nice little place, serving delicious hamburgers & handsome soldiers who played all of our favorite tunes. (By the way, what are your 3 theme songs? You didn't tell me the other evening.)
>
> Viv & I have several aches and pains from carrying our bags from train to train. Even blisters.

*Spent the evening at the Circus where we drank lemon cokes and had
fun watching the inebriates. Two sober young men (like yourself) walked us
along the lake and showed us how beautiful it looks in the evening. (Golly,
the people here certainly are friendly; never a dull moment.) Tried to learn a
few new jitterbug steps at the Victory Ballroom.*

*Intend to swim all day today and acquire a dark tan. Will be so dark
when we get back that you won't recognize us. Monday night I understand
is pretty dull. Will probably go bicycling, motorboat riding and to the Circus
in the evening.*

*Another thing Viv & I will have to do tomorrow is prepare our own
meals. Boy will we have fun. (2 beginners)*

*Viv already is in bed, but jumps out every 5 minutes with a cramp in her
toes. Think I'll have to doctor them.*

*Tis rather late and almost time to get up for breakfast. Think I'll put in,
will not sleep by the wall, though, Viv insists, first come, first served.*

Am being very good and having lots of fun. Miss you already.

Love,

Trude

*P.S. I am taking very good care of Trude for you so you needn't worry.
Golly, the bed is awful hard; we might have done better on a park bench in
the rain.—Vivian*

The dance pavilion at Lake Lawn had been renamed something
patriotic as many places were for the war. The Circus to which she
referred was a nightclub. I got a postcard that was dated the same day
with a photo of the Victory Ballroom, and the note:

Monday noon

Dear Dick,

*Will be in our cottage in about an hour. Quite cool today, but will go
swimming regardless.*

*Incidentally, what was the reason for the 50 cent I.O.U.? Was very sur-
prised to find it.*

Had much fun at "The Victory" last evening. (ballroom on other side.)

See you soon,

Trude

Of course I responded as soon as I got her letter:

Tuesday nite

6 p.m.

My Dearest Trude,

Your letter was welcomed immensely—also the card. I didn't think I would hear from you so soon, since I know that you are busy doing something all the time. Nevertheless, I was glad you hadn't forgotten your promise to write promptly.

From the contents of your masterpiece, I guess you have been having a swell time. It must be wonderful up there—dancing, swimming, and loafing. I wish I could be there enjoying that vacation paradise with you. Maybe we'll go up together some day? You know, after we're married, etc.

I suppose you won't want to leave the place after a week, but don't forget our date next Sunday nite. I wouldn't want to go alone and I would be awfully disappointed if you weren't home in time to keep the date.

You asked in the card you sent what the 50 cents was for. Well, if you recall, you paid your own way to the show the other night and I knew you wouldn't take any reimbursement so I put it in your purse while you were at the bar. You don't mind, do you? After all when I go out with my best gal, I don't expect her to pay for seeing a show when it's my obligation and privilege to do so. Enough for that subject and to the other which you questioned me about.

My three songs are "Miss You," "Everything I Love," and "Just Plain Lonesome." I think they suit the situation perfectly. I know that each one will remind you of poor "me" back home. When you're holding someone else's hand, pretend it's mine, but stop there!

Well, love, I guess I will say adios for a while. Write when you find the opportunity to do so, but make it soon 'cause I miss you very much. See you Sunday, right?

Love,

Dick

P.S. Tell Vivian, I hope that she keeps a good eye on you.

I was happy that she took the time in the middle of her wild vacation to write to me again the next morning:

July 7, 1942

Tuesday Morning

Dear Dick,

At breakfast now, which I prepared, coffee only, though. It's terribly hot, the coffee, I mean. Just finished last evening's dishes alone. Vivian's a little sick girl in bed.

Plan to walk in to the town of Delavan this morning for a few magazines & a song hit folio. It's a three mile hike each way. Expect to be back by noon when we'll go sunbathing. Sun is very warm today, think it will be a very warm day, hallelujah (I think). Yesterday was quite cold, poor Vivian almost froze to death last night. I just couldn't keep her warm, and I tried very hard. Just a cold number you know!

Have a 2-room cottage with 1 large bed in each room. Course we use just one. So if you'd like to visit us you're perfectly welcome. (If you don't snore. Walls aren't very soundproof.)

Had a very grand time last evening. First went to the Lake Lawn Lounge and had a marvelous time eating candy bars & mints, and Philip Morrising of course. They have a Panoram machine, which shows movies of the songs played. Enjoy this immensely. Lounge wasn't very lively at 11:30, so we traveled on to the Circus. All we drink are lemon Cokes, and got a kick out of ordering them at the bar where everyone else ordered something stronger. While there, met very nice people from Beloit and Chicago. Most people we meet seem to be from Chicago. They were more on the oldish side so we gave them the brush after their invitation to their chateau across the lake.

Came across our friend, Richard, Rick for short, whom we met at the pier while swimming yesterday noon. Also his friend Bob, (from Madison, Wisc.), who completed his __ years of medicine. He was very nice, more than I can say about Rick, a law student (from Oak Park). Had them down to the cottage after 1:30 when the Circus Bar closed for the evening. All we could offer them were dill pickles. Didn't have another thing in the house besides potatoes & water. Were having a very enjoyable time, as boisterous as ever, when 3 other kids came along and joined the party. A merrier group I have never seen. Didn't last very long for 2 watchmen came to our door and quieted us down. At 3 they left, but we were on their black list because of our "cold" hospitality, they said. We didn't give a hoot though, laughed it off.

Hope I didn't bore you with my Monday experiences. Are going dancing this evening to the Victory Ballroom, where Ace Brigode is furnishing the music.

Miss your everyday, twice-a-day calls, very much. Write soon.

Will have to relate tomorrow. Going to town now.

Love,

Trude

P.S. If you do come down, bring an iron and a portable. Viv wants the iron, I the portable. If you can't procure them, don't care. (Only kidding.)

Will be back early Sunday morning, we think.

Obviously she was having a good time. I was a little worried if perhaps she was having too good a time! She had apparently been smoking more cigarettes on this trip, which explains her cute reference to "Phillip Morrising." The "portable" to which she referred was a radio. She didn't own one, but always liked to have music playing and to move to the latest tunes.

She wrote to me again to tell me how much fun she was having. If there was any way I could have gotten the time off work to go up there, I would have. Not only for the fun I'm sure I would have had, but also to keep a jealous eye on Trude.

Wednesday

3 a.m.

Dear Dick,

Thinking of you. At this time I'll bet you'll be in bed. Or are you?

Had a very exciting day yesterday. Just got in, rather early, don't you think. Why you and I get in later.

After breakfast at 11:00 started hiking to town of Delavan. Walked about 10 minutes, after which we received a ride. Purchased cards & souvenirs, one for you also. Bought a genuine leather cigarette case for myself to replace the old black one Viv & I lost Sunday night. (dreary evening Sunday, it rained) Your souvenir is a surprise. After shopping an hour, our friend, Richard, (met 3 Richards already) (none as nice as you) drove us around the Lake & showed us the points of interest. Have a date Thursday at 9 a.m. to go boating & fishing with him. Grand person.

Following lunch we went swimming and swam & sunned for 4 hours. Didn't burn, but tanned. Will be brown before Saturday. Met 2 very interesting chaps on the pier. Fortunate we, they had the only portable on the pier. Heard Glenn Miller and Woody Herman (thought of you. Very often do, anyway). Had music all afternoon, goody goody. Not very much of that except at the snack, the Circus, of the ballrooms, which we don't frequent until the evening.

After swimming did our own breakfast & lunch dishes, ambitious people, and had our evening meal. Viv finally procured an iron. Our very kind neighbors were very generous with theirs. Viv pressed her clothes nicely. My turn came, and after pressing awhile forgot I had the iron on and burned a hole in my new white blouse. Handy Andy.

After that, prepared to go out. At 10:30 arrived at the Victory ballroom. Coked & danced a couple of hours & traveled to the Circus, the bright spot on the grounds. Met new friends who kidded us about drinking cokes. The bartenders are very good friends of ours now (Gene, Gus and Ivan the terrible). After 1 a.m. the players in Ace Brigode's Orch. came to the bar. Met 2 of them, Harold & George with whom we have a swimming date Wednesday noon. Very nice indeed. After their stay here, they're going on to Niles, Mich. for a while.

Jim & Scotty, friends we met Monday at the Circus, escorted us home. No party tonight. Are going bicycling Wednesday at 9:00 a.m. (Viv's going to bed now, very tired.) They're both from Chicago. Sunday, the Chez Paree (I think) & the Panther Room very nice, but recommended better places than the Chez Paree (more or less for gambling he said). The Camellia Room at the Drake, the Empire Room and the Walnut Room were his suggestions. Learning a few things about Chicago every day from these Chicagoans. Another thing, a large number of the Chez Paree patrons are Jews...I knew you'd like that.

Needn't bring an iron, just a radio. It needn't be a portable. We love music at mealtime. Can't eat in the hotel dining room daily.

I hope my experiences interest you. Don't know of anything else to write. Have you finished your book yet? Still working hard, as ever, I presume. I'm resting for both of us, so you needn't worry. Anything exciting happen to you or your friends or the city? We're having such a wonderful

time, I think I'll hate leaving. Would like to stay over Saturday & Sunday,
the liveliest nights of the week. Can't of course, would rather be with you
Sunday. Miss you. Can't wait.

>*Love,*
>*Trude*

The Coke to which she referred was still the soft drink kind; she may have been a young party girl, but wild partying in those days meant staying up listening to music and laughing until 3 a.m. The Chez Paree was one of our favorite places to go in Chicago, when we could afford the time and money to go there. The comment about the Jews was not Trude being anti-Semitic. She was anything but. She also knew how I felt on the subject so that was her way of telling me what a jerk this guy was to have said that. So even while she was waving all of these guys in front of my face, she was still saying she liked me best.

In contrast to her fun-filled days, my reply sounded a little pathetic and as though I was feeling sorry for myself, which I'm sure I was.

>*Wednesday, July 8th*
>*Dear Trude,*

At the present, I am doing exactly nothing, except writing to the one I love. Glenn Miller is on the radio now and his soothing music enables me to think of the nicest things to say to you, but I would need a book to state them all, so I'll omit them this time.

From your second letter, I guess you are having a better time than had been anticipated. Well, I hope you have a good time, but, of course, I would like to have you come home in the same state of mind (concerning you & me) that persisted before you left. If you aren't careful, you'll forget about me— "Out of sight, out of mind." Let's hope that proverb doesn't prevail in our case.

Since you've gone I have been a good boy—I mean, young man. Russ and I went to the show Tuesday nite along with Art Lennon and spent evenings at home Sunday & Monday. Of course, Russ has been prompting me to get a date, but I told him it was no use since my heart was at Lake Lawn, with you, and not in Joliet.

Whether you know it or not, you were nearly minus a boy-friend. Yesterday while I was working at my sister's home, I tripped and fell down some stairs, about 12 in number, and just about broke my neck. I wrenched a back muscle, received a slight bruise on my forearm, and was scared out of my wits. I think I shook for about 30 minutes after the accident but I am now fully recovered. The worst thing that happened was that I knocked a bucket-full of water down the stairs and got the carpeting soaked and spotted. I hope there will be no stain left, since the carpet throughout the house is worth plenty and to mar the appearance of it right at the front entrance would just about kill my sister. She's trying to keep the joint spic and span, and then I pull a stunt like that. Boy, what a jerk I am!

Well, that's the sob story for tonite. At the end of your letter, you stated that you wanted a portable and an iron. Well, I've got the iron, but no portable. Nevertheless, I am a cook ranked as the best in the Zalar household, and since you & Vivian aren't very experienced at the position I thought maybe you would need a good man like me. If you have any trouble, let me know. I am well-schooled on the art of housecleaning, etc and can furnish some suggestions.

I seem to be at a loss for words so I better close. Say hello to Vivian for me and remain being a good girl. I hope you'll write soon and the next Sunday is getting here slow but sure.

All my love,

Dick

Once again I was going for the sympathy vote with the "doing exactly nothing" comment and the story of almost dying while she was off laughing and playing with her many men in Lake Lawn. She had certainly come out of her shell since high school, and I could just imagine the stir she and Viv were creating and the way they reveled in it as they teased all those guys.

Thursday

July 9

Hello again,

Received your letter yesterday. Will definitely be back in time for our date Sunday evening. What time? It will be the only reason for coming back.

Wouldn't miss it for any Lake Lawn vacation.

Having more fun each day. Yesterday hiked to town again, or shall I say ride. After on the road 5 minutes we received a ride. Shopped for an hour & our friends waited for us and brought us back. On our return discovered we were neighbors. Ate at Delaney's yesterday noon. Very good food. Sunned again yesterday noon, for a short time only. Clouds drove us home. Had time to do dishes before our evening meal. Went bicycling at 7:00 with Jim and Scotty, 2 friends staying at Harmony Cottage across the lake. Visited their abode. Very comfortable, having all the modern conveniences which we do not. After bicycling went on to the Chateau, a beautiful dine & dance place. Boy did we swing it. Had 4 lemon cokes, nothing stronger. On our way up, we passed "Chickville" having a very large population of 8. Jim said the last time he went by it was 32, but it decreased considerably in 3 days. Lucky morticians. At the Chateau, after dancing a very fast polka number which made me very dizzy & weak, I became very sick and had to go home. At 11:00 too, it was maddening. Feel fine today, though. Will make up for it this evening.

This morning we didn't keep our boating date. Vivian was too tired, and it looked like rain. It's clearing up now, but we won't go swimming this noon. Going rollerskating instead. The rink is ¾ of a mile down the road. Nice hike. Leaving in about 10 minutes. Just Viv & I.

Going horseback riding this evening at 7:00, and dancing later, I really love it. Would rather dance with you than anyone here, you know.

Expect to get back sometime Sunday noon. Expect to go to St. Andrew's church here Sunday early. Will call you upon arrival. Will be very sorry to leave here. Time certainly does fly. Just 2 days more. Hate housekeeping though.

"Miss you" "Everything I Love" "Just Plain Lonesome"

Trude

Trude could not resist the little undertaker humor since her father was one. And in the last line she listed the titles to her three favorite songs, which also just happened to express her mood.

Neither Trude nor I were part of the "in" crowd in high school, so we were both kind of new at the dating and socializing scene, although Trude seemed to be learning fast. I wished every day to have her come home, back to me. Her descriptions of the day's events were just to drive me crazy, and I always did wonder if she kissed any of those other fellas. I never wanted to ask her in case I might not like the answer. She was always a very independent girl, and although she teased me a lot, I knew I wasn't going to be able to stop her from doing whatever she wanted to.

Thursday nite

6:30 p.m.

Dearest Trude:

Boy, you sure are prompt. I have received a letter Tuesday, Wednesday and Thursday (also two cards) and each one more informative than the previous one. Nevertheless, I still appreciate your taking the time to write every day when I know you could be doing more important things.

Nothing new has occurred in this fair metropolis since you've departed. Everything is still running smoothly, I guess at the high school and I guess Mr. Coyle is still thinking of his dear secretary at play while he is hard at work. I'll have to call him and inform him that you are having a wonderful time with the boys and the other interesting things which Lake Lawn provides to the lonesome girls who travel there from many points of the state. I only hope that my girl isn't too lonesome for me and indulges in the extra-curricular activity (which is readily undertaken beneath the moon and stars, and on a beautiful beach.) and thinks that it's me whom she's caressing. One never knows what can go on 100 miles from Joliet—especially with 2 pretty girls together in an alluring spot.

Russ just called and I have to go down to the doctor's office with him. He needs me to hold his hand, I guess. I'll write tomorrow and hope to see you early Sunday, love. Call me when you arrive—provided it's after 7:00 a.m. I get up about 7:01 to do my daily push ups on Sunday morning before going to mass.

All my love,

Dick

Russ eventually had to have surgery to remove a bad kidney, which cost him his scholarship to North Carolina State, but also kept him out of the draft. You almost felt a little embarrassed to be out wandering around without a uniform on. Especially in Chicago, guys our age were looked at a little oddly for not being in the service.

I made sure I answered her, letter for letter. I didn't want her to forget about my pitiful pining back in Joliet.

> *July 10, 1942*
>
> *Dear Trude,*
>
> *Hi dear! Well, your got another day of freedom before you return to the clutches of the future Doc Zalar. Disgusting, isn't it? Our date for this Sunday is still intact, I see, by your last letter. Tonight is Friday and in Joliet, that means date night, but your little boy is going to the show unchaperoned. I think Russ has his usual date with JoAnn, so I'll have to scout around and see what I can scare up around the neighborhood.*
>
> *It is hotter than ____ today. I worked pretty hard and now I am ready for a shower. The temperature hit about 90 and I was drenched with perspiration. I got a little burnt, but nothing to speak of. I suppose it is warm there the majority of the time and everybody receives a tan without much trouble. I do hope I can recognize you when you return. By your letters, you must look like a negro.*
>
> *I was very sorry to hear you were ill the other day. Too much night life, no doubt or maybe something else. I hope you have fully recovered by now or else your last few days won't be very enjoyable.*
>
> *It is now 6:25 p.m. and the train will take this letter to Chicago at 7, so I'll close and see you soon. Say hello to Viv and the other boys.*
>
> *Love,*
>
> *Dick*

She told me every detail of her man-filled days in the sun, but she signed her letters "Love, Trude," so I was never quite sure if I had anything to worry about or not.

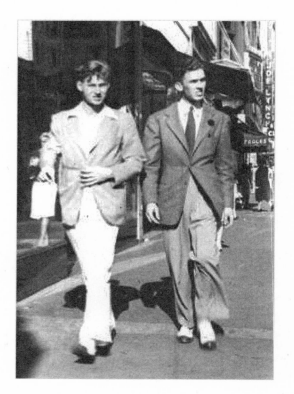

Joe Limacher and me. Two
dapper gents on the town in San
Francisco. (top)

Me in front of Joe DiMaggio's
restaurant in San Francisco.

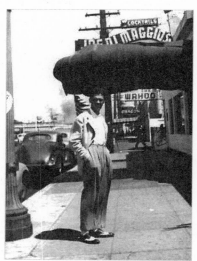

Changing Jobs, Changing Schools

Trude came back to me, and our dating resumed. She had been employed at the high school since October of 1940, and her weekly pay was not all that great. When the war came, a variety of job opportunities became immediately available at better wages. During August of 1942 she advised Mr. Coyle (Dale Dudley, as she liked to call him) she would be leaving.

Like many other people, she decided to get a job with a defense contractor, and she found a position at the Elwood Ordnance Plant where Russ and I had worked during the summer of 1941. Starting pay for laborers that year was 90 cents an hour—quite good wages. We took the jobs for the money, even though we understood the risk. Although our jobs had nothing to do with the making of munitions, just being that close to them posed some danger. Russ and I mainly found ourselves digging foundations. I wasn't really cut out for strenuous manual labor, unlike Russell, who was a good enough athlete to have earned a basketball scholarship to the North Carolina State University. At 145 pounds I was a bit too scrawny for the work, but the pay was too good to turn down. We got a raise when the job got even harder—unloading boxcars full of heavy crates of sewer tiles. It made guys like Russ stronger; I thought it was going to kill me.

The danger of the plant was driven home to everyone in the area the year after we worked there, when, on June 5, 1942, the night stillness of Joliet was shattered just after 2 a.m. The sound and reverberations of a powerful explosion traveled the 15 miles from the plant up the riverbed of the Des Plaines, which runs just west of town on its way to the Mississippi, hundreds of miles south. Once people realized what had happened, the fright was unbelievable. Some explosives being assembled at the plant had accidentally detonated, blowing a hole in the ground 26 feet deep and large enough to accommodate six rail cars. The next day's paper carried the terrible toll: 21 dead and 35 wounded or missing; windows throughout the complex were shattered. It scared everyone who worked there or lived in the area and made all of the employees quite jumpy for a while, but the war work had to go on.

With her secretarial skills and her ability to deal with people, Trude was hired by the Fire and Safety division of DuPont at the plant. Again there was some bit of risk, but Trude accepted it. Her salary was $25 for five and a half days a week, which was a major improvement over her pay at the school, and it had her working with adults instead of feeling like she was still in high school. She also felt as though she could contribute a little something to the war effort, which most people felt obligated to do. She learned the job's needs quickly and soon fell into a new and more stimulating routine. She was chosen to be photographed along with senior members of the company for an ad for the division.

Her biggest obstacle with her job was transportation. She had no car, and the bus ride was long and inconvenient. On occasions she was late for work, and she knew that couldn't keep happening, so although she liked the work itself, she was quickly looking for another job.

As the summer was winding down, Joe Limacher and I took a train trip to California; it was my first major excursion out of Illinois since my sister Vida and I traveled to Texas when I was 12. We visited San Francisco and Los Angeles, staying with some relatives of his part of the time. It was great to get out and see some of the world and began my attachment to the Golden State, which would bring me back there many times over the course of my life.

After my third year in college at Champaign, I had enough credits to enter medical school. I was admitted to the Chicago branch of the University of Illinois in September of 1942. Again, I roomed in a fraternity house, a six-block walk to the medical campus, since to find a place to live in the neighborhood was not very easy and a little dangerous for a small-town "hick." There were stories of students being mugged at gun or knifepoint, which made me want to be cautious whenever I went out at night.

Trude and I resumed our correspondence even though Chicago was much closer than Champaign. Writing was still the easiest way to communicate, even though I came home as often as I could catch a ride with someone. Phone calls even from Chicago were more than I could afford. She still teased me and kept me on my toes. She was never going to let me take her for granted.

She had started coming into Chicago once or twice a week to do some shopping and would usually call me and sometimes have dinner with me or at least see me for a little while before she had to take the train or bus back to Joliet. On some of these trips, she would end up riding the last bus at midnight which would get her to Joliet about 1 a.m. She would have to take a cab home, and then have to get up early for work the next day. She always seemed to have a lot more energy than I did.

In her work as a secretary, she used Gregg shorthand, which she and many other girls had studied in high school business classes. Taking rapid dictation was a very marketable job skill, and sometimes she would write a few words or a sentence or sometimes cover an entire page of one of her letters with strange squiggles. She'd reeled her thoughts off, but left me at a loss as to what she had written. She teased me with this, and I could hardly wait to talk to her on the phone or get another letter that might explain it. Or sometimes she'd make me wait until the next date. She kept me at my wits' end. I had been back at school almost a month when she added a special code to the end of a letter:

Wednesday, September 30

Dear Dick,

I hope you are feeling better than I am today. Feeling very weak & ill, so ill that a date with Viv had to be broken for this evening. Mom said, "It's not surprising, with all the rest you've been getting. You aren't made of iron

75

you know, at that pace you couldn't survive more than two years." I tried to explain, but it was useless. Incidentally, she knew the time I came in Saturday morning. She mentioned it the other night and wondered if we were celebrating your last few days home. This being the occasion, she didn't reprimand me too strongly.

Received your letter today. Hope you aren't studying too hard. It's 8 p.m. now, the time we'd be stepping out; but I don't mind staying in, we'll make up for it this weekend. I'm being good & can't wait to see the surprise you have for me. I have one for you, too.

Today Viv asked me how often I write to you. When I informed her four times a week she exclaimed, "I wonder if I will ever get it that bad?" Need I explain? Her statement I mean. Doesn't it confirm something I reiterated several times many evenings?

The men in the office were teasing George about having to ask Alice whether or not he could join in the crap game scheduled for an evening next week. He said, "Gee, I still haven't paid the $5 for the party last week." Rayburn should talk, telling other men how to get around their wives when he can't handle his, she tells him what to do.

Purchased a new frame for your picture. Looks very neat on the dresser now.

Tomorrow is payday again. That means another charm. This one is going to be a golf bag and clubs, numbering 11 charms in all.

Will see you on Saturday evening. Remember I'll love you always and miss you very much.

Lots of love,

Trude

As the postscript she included a sentence in Gregg shorthand. Then translated it for me:

P.S. I love you very much, always will, remember.

This remained our code for the rest of our correspondence, and for our whole relationship, in fact.

Of course, I had to respond in some way, and I selected a few phrases in German. I had studied it for four years and I could still remember a good bit. She had no idea what I said, but after I had given her the translation, it served as our second "code" and the P.S. signoffs in our letters.

Things had moved along so quickly during the summer that after I was back at school and missing her, I decided I wanted more. We wrote a few times a week and saw each other on weekends as time allowed. My studies suffered a bit, I'm sure, between the time spent writing to her, the time spent running home to visit her, and the times when I found myself just staring into space and thinking about her—when last I was with her, when I would see her again—instead of staring at the books. I started pressing her to get married, but she kept trying to put off the date, at least until I was done with school.

I wrote her a letter to which I added my own secret message:

November 9, 1942

My dearest Trude,

I received your swell letter this afternoon and it sort of gave me an idea to come home more often than I do. When I do come home on Saturdays, I wish that we could be together all the time, but I guess we'll have to wait for the 3 years to pass. You consider shortening the time, would you? I wish you would, because I miss you terribly when I am up here in school. During Xmas vacation, we'll have to go out every night, if that's all right with you.

Seems as if the class on Monday is always dull. Everyone is just about half asleep and I find it very difficult to keep my eyes open, half the time. (School isn't very interesting, so I'll stop here.)

I love you very, very much sweetie, and I know nothing will ever come between us. I wouldn't hurt you for the world and if I was a millionaire, I'd buy you the world with a fence around it. I am awfully sorry for getting so worked up when you say things that tease me, but I get so jealous when they do arise that I don't know how to control myself. You understand, don't you, honey?

I have a test tomorrow in anatomy so I'll have to start pounding the books. I hope I can hit it, because all of the grades I get from now on will count for or against me. I'll write tomorrow nite.

All my love and kisses,

Dick

P.S. Ich liebe dich meine schone Frau. Mein lieb ist sehr grosze. Ich geben eine tausend kusze.

I wrote to her again the next night and again included the code at the end.

Tuesday nite

My dearest Trude:

Yours truly is one sad boy today. I expected a letter, but when I rushed to the mail-box, there was none to be found. Maybe be it will be here tomorrow morning. Anyway, I hope so. I like to hear from you very much, as I've told you many times already, and no letter during the day is very discouraging.

We didn't have an exam today as was expected. I studied till 1 last night but I didn't absorb too much so I guess it was better that we didn't get one. Maybe tomorrow will be the day of reckoning. I have a make-up test Friday in anatomy so I'll have to study quite hard for it.

If you have any news about Faulkner's dates, would you let me know in one of your letters? He is quite hard up for a girl. I guess nobody likes him— of course, I'm only kidding but he never seems to find the right girl. I know he envies me, because I've got the nicest and sweetest girl in Joliet. So he'll have to take all the second rate girls or else go to a different town and find the top one there. Poor kid—right?

I've got to close now, sweetie, be good and take care of yourself. I'll be writing tomorrow night.

All my love and kisses,

   Dick

P.S. Ich liebe dich sehr grosze, meine schone Frau. Alle meinen Lieb ist dich.

I had asked Trude to try to find a date for my friend Jim Faulkner, who never seemed to have much luck on his own. Of course I would no longer go cruising for girls with him as we did when I missed out on Bank Night at the movies.

November 10, 1942

Dear Dick:

Please convey my regrets to Faulkner for I am very very sorry that I cannot do the immense favor he asks of me. Not knowing the girls very intimately, I would feel a little ridiculous asking to reserve a date for him. Perhaps, I am little backward for feeling as I do, but I do not think it would be proper for me to do as he asks. When I was born it is true I was clothed in as many clothes as Cupid, but I was not endowed with the arrow. In the excitement and confusion, the arrow was forgotten or mislaid. Fancy that! Something (a favor) smaller, I would be very glad to do, but not this. Think it's absurd. I suggest that he write, or call. Money doesn't mean anything to him, does it?

You had better learn your bones and muscles, etc, for there is the future to consider. About shortening the time of 3 years, I don't think it's wise. It really should be lengthened, don't you think? Going out every night during Xmas vacation is 100% yes (ok) with me, but you have your health to think about. 10 hours rest every night means retiring at about 11:00. Even George thinks you should rest more than you do. Don't ask me how he knows just how long you do rest. He probably knows your family. Another thing, you must step out on Sunday nights if you have difficulty keeping your eyes open Monday afternoon. Right?

Mr. Vanderbilt, the world with a fence around it sounds pretty good, but I'd prefer it with the Japs and Germans excluded, leaving only peace-loving people. Better still, forget the world, I'd settle for a 2 1/2 carat diamond, (huge, isn't it?) and you. One of the girls we ride with is going down to Illinois to attend the Military Ball, a week from next Friday, Nov. 20, I believe. (her friend is a freshman). Lucky girl! A couple of days before gas rationing starts too. Offered to let her wear one of my formals, if it appeals to her. Perhaps in the future, I can wear one of hers. We're discussing pet-ting, and the like, this afternoon. Ethel brought up the subject by telling us her sister who disapproves of it, and thinks it horrid. "She won't even let anyone kiss her goodnite," Ethel said. I interposed, "I feel as she does, my friend and I never pet." George came back with, "I'll bet you and your boyfriend get so wrapped up in each other that you can't tell who's who." I wonder how he knows. He hit the nail right on the head didn't he? He was just teasing me, and he loves to do that. Good guess, though.

Met one of the girls from school today. Gee, I miss the place; I liked it so. The school kids and fellow workers, and Coyle and Skeel and everybody. Don't have time to stop in to see them either. Think I'll go to the Junior

College play Friday. Might bump into some of the kids. But I miss you a lot more than I do the kids, in a different way, of course. I love you very, very, very, very much. Again, again, again, again & again. Glad today is Tuesday, which means that I'll see you in a short time. Hope school isn't too difficult. Hate to see or hear that you have to study &study & study. (No, mother didn't break a lot of records before I was born.) Look forward to your letters & enjoy them tremendously.

Goodnite sweetie, will write tomorrow.

Lots of love,

Trude

It's funny now to read how even serious kissing or petting were considered risqué, and only the worst kind of guy would try to go further than that, and only the lowest kind of girl would let him.

I so much enjoyed Trude's letters and the tiny little details of her life that let me get to know her better. I was gaga enough over her to want to know everything she did. I guess my studies were getting me down, and as I said, I wasn't the best student and seemed to have to work twice as hard as everyone else to keep up. A letter from Trude was often the only bright spot of my day. I guess I was also a little insecure as to whether Trude was going to wait for me to come home each week. Trude wrote back promptly.

Wednesday

November 11, 1942

Dear Dick,

I cannot understand what happened to my Monday nite letter. I mailed it before going to work as I usually do. Perhaps Russell came upon it at the post office and took it out to write another of his love notes to you. Sorry you didn't receive it & was disappointed. You can always count on my writing, writing a few lines at least.

Perhaps this is "blowing my own horn." Pop had a TL for me this morning. He asked me to tell you that he thinks I am one of the nicest girls he's ever met and a prize like me you should hang on to. "I'm an old man," he said, "and I've met plenty." How's that? Now I hate more than ever telling him I'm going to change riders. But I will.

Had another brainstorm today. Ethel and I were reprimanded for leaving the office at 4:58 yesterday. We had a chip on our shoulders all day and I was thinking seriously of leaving the great organization. I intend to attend comptometer school & try to get a job at Public Service, working 5 days a week. Won't that be wonderful? You're probably thinking it's a great fuss over nothing, but that's only one thing. The boss is so irritable lately that we're afraid to go the washroom to wash our hands. It doesn't bother me as much as it does the other girls for I'm just anxious to get "fired" and work elsewhere. Perhaps, Chicago!

Love,

Trude

P.S. All right, don't keep me in the dark. Translate the Greek!

Just as Trude had tormented me with the shorthand, I hadn't translated my German code for her. Eventually I did. The first one meant, "I love you my beautiful lady. My love is very great. I give you a thousand kisses." And the second German P.S. was something similar. "Pop" was a man who worked with both Trude and me at the Elwood Plant. He lived in Joliet and was often Trude's ride to work when gas rationing, weather, the car not working or other calamities didn't prevent him from driving. On those mornings she had a long walk into downtown Joliet to catch the bus for a long ride to the plant which meant she'd be quite late. A "TL" was her little code for a "Tender Loving"—in other words a compliment or sweet thing.

Some of Trude's letters in November, 1942, started arriving with penciled notes written on the envelopes. The first one said:

Hello you jerk. What's cooking? Hows school? I'm watching Trude for you. That is if she needs it. Praise the Lord and Pass the Ammunition.

Russ

Russ had gotten a part-time job sorting mail at the post office after he recovered from his surgery. I had done this as a Christmas job myself a couple times. Russ had apparently seen one of her letters to me come through and decided to add his own little note. I also noticed that where she had addressed it to "Mr. Richard W. Zalar," he had added "Esq." Later that month, he got hold of another of her letters and added a pencil note:

Well, well, here I am again. How are they hangin? Swell. I miss you so much my darling. I can hardly wait till we go out smooching again—you big man. Remember till the flowers bloom again—

Guess who

Then he added other little notes on the envelopes including Nuts to you, V for Victory, and Remember Pearl Harbor. On the address, he again added an Esq. to my name and added the words "rat trap" after the name of my fraternity house. Another of his exterior notes said:

Well goo-goo eyes, what's new? Do you still love me, I hope so as you know I love you. Oh dear, there I go again spilling the beans. But you should understand how I feel with my hands.

Trudy Pisut

From Old Dubuque

There was a column in the newspaper that used to regularly carry letters signed "from old Dubuque," so Russ was making reference to that little local joke. And the final note I got from him was:

Oh look it's me again. I'm going to Billings today so I'll give you a buzz on the phone as I miss your charming voice. I love you so much my darling. It seems years since we smooched & did other things—

Trude Pisut

Old Dubuque

I told him I should have him arrested for tampering with the US mail. Russ didn't last long at the post office, not because of his tampering, but because the bending and lifting was too hard on him after the operation. I went from one day enjoying his jokes to the next getting a shock from Trude. In one letter she went from an amazing opening line to shattering my world:

Sunday

November 15, 1942

Dearest Dick,

Could there be another you? Could anyone take your place? Is there another perfect smile to make me feel sole rejoice? Would I be thrilled and enraptured while I listen to another voice?

Is there another loving hand, which I could hold from morning to night. And could there be a love as grand as ours, so real, so right? Can there be other lips that I may kiss thrill me like yours do? Can there be other perfectly beautiful nights and afternoons with anyone else? There's just one answer I can give, will be the same the long years through, No matter how long I might live, there will always be you, never another. (This is what I referred to this noon.)

I'm at home all alone this evening. Rather, Ag & I are. Viv backed out of going to the show this evening. I won't see "I Married an Angel" after all. Tomorrow I'm going in Chicago after work, did I tell you? Tuesday is the night I'll receive my permanent. I don't believe the above-mentioned movie will be at the Princess Wednesday, so I believe I will see it when it is at the Majestic!! (This 2nd cigarette really tastes pretty good.)

Can't think of anything to write except that to say I miss you more tonight than ever. But I found a substitute for you. It's your picture. It's so real especially that smile, guess I can wait until next Saturday when you will come home again.

Does your heart have a two-way stretch? Yes? No? If you don't get it, I'll explain.

I love you very much, dearest. More & more each day/week. Do you think we could separate for several months? Let's try it and note our reactions. I often stop and think that we are mis-mated. I cannot tell you my reasons for thinking so, but I'm almost positive I might be right. I may be wrong. Why don't we stop seeing each other and find out? I'm almost sure that in no time at all you will find someone more your type. Course this will break my heart as much as it might yours, but I'm confident (sorry) that we both have two-way stretch hearts. We're still young & love affairs like ours will eventually wear off. I can't help feeling the way I do, but you may see my side of it sometime. I don't think you should become so attached to one individual as you seem to be to me, while attending school. We seem to be so

in love, each week making our love greater, that I really do not think it wise
to get any greater. I think it is more than I can swallow. Remember, I love
you, as much as you love me, and I'm only thinking of what might be better
for both of us in the long run. It doesn't mean that we sever our relationship
permanently, but temporarily under our conditions that will be best for both
of us. Course for a while, we'll miss each other a great deal, but it's just like
anything else that we've owned a long time and have to part with. Don't
think I'll write until I've heard from you in reference to the above.

Until then,

Trude

P.S. I haven't thought about this at all today until this evening.
Truthfully, please believe me.

I sat on my bed shaking. It was as though someone else had taken possession of her. Even her signature was different—not signed on the right side of the page with "all my love..." None of our secret codes.

I stared at the page analyzing the writing. Could this really have come from my Trude?

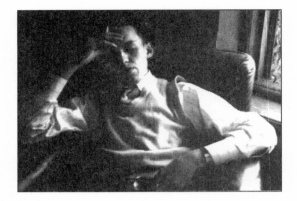

Dick, the weary
student. (top)

Trude at a foot-
ball game.

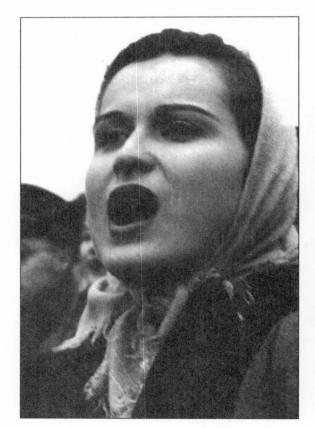

Trouble in Paradise

With shaking hand I sat down to try to write a response. My handwriting was never as neat as hers, but in this letter I ran words together and scribbled, as anxious as I was to get my words on paper. If there was any way I could have afforded a long-distance call on my very limited student budget I would have called her for an explanation.

> *SAE*
>
> *Monday Nite*
>
> *11/16/42*
>
> *My Dearest Trude,*
>
> *I just got in from playing basketball and as usual, the first place I headed for was the mailbox. But this was the day which in my estimation, the world fell in. At the present, the fellows are downstairs eating, but my stomach is on the blink after reading your letter.*
>
> *In all of my life I have never had such a shock as I got tonight. I don't know what happened yesterday, but I think I know why you wrote your letter. I'll explain when I see you Saturday.*
>
> *I suppose you think it a little silly for a fellow to shed a few tear drops, especially me, but I must admit it happened to me. I can't see how anyone could write such a letter to one with whom they are supposed to be in love. If there was any incident or causative factor that earned such a drastic move, I was ignorant of it. But I know that something happened.*
>
> *Your idea of separating for 2 or 3 months I cannot believe to be coming from you. Isn't it possible for 2 people to be in love much when the situation is the same as ours—my attending school and your working? Honey, right*

now, I don't know what to do. Funny ideas have been running through my head. One which is very prevalent at the moment is that I am going to quit school. I told you once if I told you a hundred times that I have one goal in life and that is to be your husband in the habit of a medical man, but I guess I have only one alternative now, and that is elsewhere.

I have reread your letter 4 times in the past 10 minutes and each time my heart is heavier and my idea becomes stronger. I may be a little eccentric in some respects, but when I find the right girl, I intend to keep her or life isn't worth fighting for. I know that you love me very much and I believe anything you tell me to the fullest extent. The same holds true with you. Right? (I mean when I tell you I love you, I know you believe me.)

Another subject, which I really can't understand, is your reference to our "mismating." I don't see it your way. What is the matter with me? I am not an imbecile or moron or suffering from any social exclusion. Just because I am a little forceful in asking you to do things for me doesn't mean I am trying to run your mode of life. I know that I was a little selfish in asking you to stay in during the week, but I thought that letters and our dates on the weekend would sort of make up for it. Honey, I told you that I'd do anything for you, but I can't seem to see how I could be away from you. I'm just human, you know and I've never been in love like this before.

I recall one night this summer when you told me that we were not meant for each other, but I expressed a different view point if you'll remember I thought that we had agreed on that matter a long time ago. I guess it still persists in your beautiful head.

Now you have heard my side of the story. If you want to write to me, and I hope you do, I expect an answer which will make me feel like a new man. Otherwise, I doubt whether I can change your mind. I expect to go out this Saturday with you and if nothing can be accomplished, I guess you know what will occur—good-bye to medical school.

All my love to you will grow every day till Saturday when I can be with you again. If you have time, call me when you get to Chicago.

Love,

Dick

P.S. Our code is still "ditto" and will be forever.

I sent the letter Special Delivery to make sure she got it quickly. Obviously I had been writing too many papers for medical school from the strange words I was using and the convoluted sentences. I guess I should not have expected Trude to sit home at night writing to me. In that tiny house there was no privacy of any kind so I am sure she had to escape to a soda fountain with Viv or to a movie whenever she could. I just hated the idea of guys checking her out or talking to her. I guess I was getting a little love-sick and jealous. I was new at this whole business of serious love affairs and had a lot to learn.

I was ready to get married in the fall of '42, and she was probably quite wise to apply the brakes a bit, but it felt as though she was hitting the brakes too hard and was about to launch me through the windshield. She responded the evening after she got my letter:

Tuesday 11/17/42

Dearest Dick,

Please believe me when I say I am very sorry to have upset you so by that very cruel letter of mine Sunday night. So sorry, as a matter of fact, that I'm having a little difficulty writing this letter, for my tear-filled eyes are not helping matters at all. Cannot understand myself, why I wrote it. Don't know what possessed me. I must have been serious, for I know I wasn't teasing. I think I passed that stage. I didn't really mean it, though. I believe I would have been more heartbroken than you. You say you would leave school. Please don't do that. I understand that a medical career was your ambition since about a decade ago. Giving that up would certainly be a crime which I wouldn't want to be the instigator of, (as you would say.)

I must have been feeling a little blue over something which does not concern both of us, although I can think of no plausible reason for writing the letter to alleviate the condition. Just another of my unexplainable peculiarities. Regretted it immensely after mailing it. Did not realize it would affect you as deeply or greatly as it had, but I am sure I would have been just as puzzled and surprised had I received a similar letter from you after our too-perfect weekend. Couldn't have had a more enjoyable time had I made preparations for it weeks in advance.

*Love you very, very much. Undoubtedly would feel very, very blue if we
two parted, but I always seem to be the instigator, as you would say. It certainly would be a calamity. Our relationship is nothing to be trifled with, I
am very slowly beginning to realize.*

*In your letter you state that you think you know what prompted me to
write my letter. I wonder what you're thinking. I would like to go over the
whole letter with you Saturday, so be prepared.*

*Would love to see the Notre Dame-Northwestern game. (Saturday?) Will
join you in keeping my fingers crossed.*

*Received the 44 Sunday nite kisses tonight. Mmmmm-mmmm-
mmmmm-mmmmm. Hope I can deliver mine personally, but I think I'll wait
until Saturday nite.*

*I do hope things are running smooth at school. Am very sorry to have
caused an interruption in your not-too-smooth running program. Will "look
before I leap" in the future.*

*Cannot express very clearly or adequately my sorrow for my unexplain-
able deed. Love you very dearly and couldn't think of hurting you. You are
very kind to me and I could not expect any more; it isn't humanly possible to
know anyone more thoughtful and considerate than you.*

*In reference to mismating, it wasn't you that I was thinking that didn't
measure up to certain standards or ideals, it was I. There certainly is nothing wrong with you, sweetie. Sincerely.*

*Goodnight my love. If this letter doesn't clarify all questions in your
mind, please inform. I will do my best to answer them.*

All of my love,

Trude

*P.S. I love you very, very much my ideal lover. Will be anxiously awaiting
your return. Cannot live without you, I am sure.*

She had to wait until late at night to have any sort of privacy to
write and not have to explain to so many prying siblings why she was
crying over my letters.

From her work as a secretary, Trude's writing also tended
towards formality and words that were bigger than necessary for

our love letters, and part of the stiltedness was just the way people wrote in the mid-20th century. I guess we both were taught this way in our high school composition classes.

Like me, Trude had never really been in love before, and I think the pace at which we were moving and the depths to which we were going was starting to scare us both. I knew I would rather continue on our plunge into love than try to stop the freefall—I think at this point the G-forces would have done me in. Or my father would have, if I had told him I was quitting med school for a girl! I'm not sure whether the idea of my being a doctor began with him or me, but that is all we had ever assumed I would be.

ETA of Nu Sigma Nu

626 S. Ashland Boulevard

Chicago, Ill.

November 18, 1942

My Dearest Trude,

I was very glad to hear from you today. Your letter was the most wonderful ever. I am sure glad that you did not mean what you said in your previous letter. If that would have happened (our separation), I don't know what I would have done without you. Really, I couldn't visualize not being with you for such a long time—life wouldn't be in me then.

Today, I hit the jackpot. I not only received your swell letter, but I got 88 and 97 on my 2 tests in Anatomy. Not as good as it should be, but I'll do better with your confidence behind me. Now watch me roll. Every course will be a B or better or I'll know the reason why.

Honey, you are the sweetest girl in all the world. I love you immensely and miss you very much. If I could be with you all the time, I'd be in heaven. When you say that you're not right for me, I know that isn't true. If I couldn't have you, nobody else would do and I mean that from the bottom of my heart.

Goodnight, sweetheart. Saturday is a long way off (as it always is when I'm at school) but I can wait patiently. I'm so happy tonight, I had a notion to come see you, but I guess your beautiful pictures will have to do till I see you. Bye for now. I'll write tomorrow.

Lots of love,

Dick

P.S. "Ditto" our code.

"Ditto" my German poem.

Tonite's kisses: xxxxxxxxxxxxxxxxxxxxxxxxxxxxxxxxxxxxxxxxxxxxxxxxxxx

I could get a little melodramatic at times, but she really did have me confused.

"...Or I'll know the reason why..." was a quirky little expression I had picked up meaning "or else." I wasn't implying that Trude would be the reason for my flunking out, although if she had dumped me, I might very well have dropped out or my grades would have fallen to the point they'd boot me out. Whether that might mean immediate induction to the military or my poor eyesight would spare me, I didn't know. If Trude had stopped seeing me and I flunked, I might not have cared so much about going off to be shot. Although I joked about it, too many of my friends were in uniform and might face that fate any day.

I thought Trude had put thoughts of a separation out of her head after scaring me half to death with it the first time, but when I was home one weekend in December, she again suggested we take some time off from each other—that things were just moving too fast for her. She said there was a good reason for this needed break, and then would not tell me what that reason was. She was now driving me crazy in a bad way instead of in the nice way she usually did. At times I was confused as to whether this was the same trial separation, or a new one.

December 11 1942

Friday

My sweetest Trude:

I just got in. Time being 8:30. I didn't leave the house till 7 and thought of calling you but decided not to since we had settled our dispute beforehand. If I had called, it would be just to tell you how much I care for you and how much you mean to me, but that is a known fact of 6 months standing.

I found that being away from you is terrific and makes me so very
blue, even though I had seen you 2 hours ago. Of course, I am lonely
when the days pass, but tonite has been worse than ever. I guess you
know why.

Honey, I am so mixed up that my mind is a jumble of thoughts. I've
said it before and now I say it once again, I can't visualize our separation. It
is unbelievable. It would seem very plausible if we had reasons for it. You
won't tell me yours and I don't have any so I don't know what to do or how
to make you change your attitude. If you would only tell me what hap-
pened, I think we could solve our mixup. I know the one alternative is not
our separation, but rather an answer to your deed. It can't be that bad that
you can't tell me of it. You will tell me on Saturday nite won't you, sweet-
heart? Please!!!

The week-end passed quickly but I had a swell time. I'm glad you let me
come over today, even though we talked about matters which hurt me very
much. Just your presence makes me feel good and I do hope I can see you
every Sat. nite and Sunday afternoon from now till that day we are mar-
ried. Bye.

All my love & kisses,

Dick

P.S. I love you so very much words can't express it.

P.S. our motto: "Try to keep us together."

I used "terrific" in the old sense of being filled with terror, not the
way it is usually used today meaning "good." I didn't even wait for
Trude to answer before my anxiety got the better of me and I had to
write to her again:

December 12, 1942

Saturday

My sweetest Trude:

Today, I was pondering as to the status of our plight.

Sometimes I feel that I am entirely to blame for everything. I don't
know what I have done in the past 6 months to cause a disruption of our
relationship but I am sure I haven't treated you the way I should. Maybe I

*don't deserve such a girl as sweet as you. Only you can decide that. Will it
be a positive answer in January? I hope so very, very much.*

*I am pretty sick this evening. My cold has progressed to a feverish state
and I feel like I did the time of my last illness. I'm going to the hospital for
an x-ray the first chance I get and find out if I am ok inside. My Dad
severely reprimanded me for not taking care of myself but I told him I was
unable to avoid the cold even though I have kept myself bundled up when
outside. Sanitarium here I come.*

*Thursday is the last exam day of this quarter. I have been studying pretty
hard for it so I should do better than I did in my first exam. (47—wow)!*

*I sure feel blue, honey. Even though you agreed to try to prevent our
breaking-up, I have a funny feeling inside of me, one that has never been
there before. It feels as if something is being pulled out by its roots never to be
replaced by anything. Sweetheart, if you can see your way clear to continue
our steady life I would be the happiest fellow in the world. That would be an
ideal Xmas gift for me—nothing else would have to be added.*

*Bye for now, darling. I love you above anything in this world and to be
away from you for a week leaves me with a terrific anxiety to be with you.*

All my love and kisses,

Dick

P.S. Our code-forever!! Right?

P.S. My newest song: "Do you care?"

I found a song title that expressed how I felt. She wrote right back
trying to explain things, but I knew I would have to see her again
before I felt really reassured.

12/15/42

Tuesday

Dearest Darling Dick,

*How is that cold of yours? I do hope it's gone. I would abhor going to
the hospital daily during your Xmas vacation. Please take care of that nasty
cold, just for me. Mine is practically gone. It was pretty bad today; I cried all
day long & was sorry I didn't stay home. Feel lots better now though. I
believe it was that inhalant that was given to me that did the trick. Please
try to do away with yours.*

Received both your letters today. Did you know you're two days late? That is both letters are misdated, your Sunday letter dated the 11th & the other dated the 12th.

I noticed that in your letters you elaborate on the occurrence of Sunday noon. I thought we were going to forget it and not discuss it further, for I thought everything was settled. I can readily see why it is almost impossible to dismiss it from our minds completely. It really seems to involve two lives. I am living up to my promise of doing my best, but I cannot tell you the reason for the suggested separation. No matter how great your appeal, I cannot weaken and tell you. I know it doesn't seem fair, but that is how it will have to be. I'm very sorry that I can't confide in you in regard to this matter; it is the one and only situation that I cannot mention. Sorry dearest.

I, too, had a very pleasant weekend. I didn't intend to hurt you Sunday noon, but was something that had to be discussed sooner or later. It was a very distasteful task as far as I was concerned, but there were very sincere feelings involved. I was just as upset as you, if not more, for I do love you very much and a separation from you is something that I hoped never would happen. It does sound mysterious, but I am doing my best to right things, that is, "Trying to keep us together."

You seem to shoulder all censure or guilt for the pending catastrophe. Dearie, it isn't any deed or action of yours that motivated the incident of Sunday noon. Putting the shoe on the other foot, it no doubt was something that I had done, which is true. It seems serious enough to make me feel very guilty, so guilty that I am not deserving of as nice & sweet a friend as you.

Please try to rid yourself of that pessimistic attitude in reference to our future. Believe me when I say I'm doing my best. I love you so much that I'd do anything in my power to make you happy, not only for the present, but for always. A person who has shown as much kindness, interest, and thoughtfulness as you have certainly cannot be passed up and forgotten as easily as a crammed lesson.

Love you very much dearest, and you can count on my thinking of your welfare and future before mine in anything that I do or intend to do. If we do have the good fortune of pairing-up for always, you will not regret it, for

I will be the best partner anyone has ever had or hoped for. I will put forth
all efforts to measure up to this near-perfection.

Goodnight my one & only. Please take care of yourself, just for me. Love
you much & don't want anything to occur that will interfere with your
plans. Miss you very very much, and am anxiously awaiting your return
next Saturday. Think of you constantly.

Lots of love, Always,

Trude

P.S. I love you. Our "code."

2 P.S. Yes I do care, very much, dearie.

Thanks again for the flowers, very beautiful.

I had thought of a million reasons why she was going through this
and couldn't tell me. What did she have to feel guilty about? Had she
kissed another guy—or worse? Had she heard some sort of false
rumors about me that made her distrust me, and then didn't want to
reveal the source since it was someone close to me? Did she hear what
my sister and some of my friends has said about her being from the
wrong side of town and she didn't want to drive a wedge by telling
me who said what? What could her reason be? But she did refer to
"our future."

Did we still have one?

December 15, 1942

My sweetest Trude:

I got your letter this morning and it sure encouraged me. In fact, it was
so wonderful, I feel as if nothing had happened Sunday. Is it all right if I
assume your actions as kidding ones? I hope so, honey.

Did you get my flowers last nite? I had originally told my aunt to send
them Tuesday and when you said yesterday was the 14th, I nearly dropped
over in the telephone booth. One of the fellows misled me in saying that
Monday was the 13th when I asked him. Our anniversary had been on my
mind for the past few weeks that I figured I wouldn't get the dates mixed. As
soon as I finished talking to you, I called Joliet and asked my aunt to send
the flowers at once. She said she would, so I hope you got them on this most
important day of my life.

I was expecting a surprise you sent this afternoon, but I guess it won't be here till tomorrow. I also have one for you. It's just a small gift but expresses my deep love for you.

Just think in 4 days I'll be home for two weeks. Wow! Nothing to worry about (I mean school etc.), except your decision on our affair.

Well, darling I have to hit the books. What a pain in the neck they are. The more I study, the less I know. Pitiful, isn't it?

I love you very much, honey. Miss you twice as much. Hope you feel the same. Bye for now.

All my love & kisses,

Dick

Our code—forever and ever.

P.S. My new song is... "There are such things."

Our daily letters often crossed in the mail with the responses to questions posed several letters ago. Most of the time we tried to write daily although it was not always possible with school, work, and other obligations. But we had come to depend so much on each other's letters to brighten our days, that not getting any mail would depress whichever one of us was let down.

12/16/42

Wednesday

Dearest darling Dick,

By the time you receive this letter your last final will be completed and you will be walking on air again. I am so glad that you will have a great deal of leisure time. Then, maybe, you can give me a little thought now & then.

I did not receive a letter from you today. No doubt, the beginning of the Christmas rush has delayed your letter. Was informed that the mail carrier was later than usual today, and made only one trip. Might receive two letters tomorrow, I hope.

Am going out tonight. Am getting in trim for next week, when I'll, no doubt, step out twice or three times instead of once. Will be good, though, as you requested. Am going just to be doing something. You understand, don't you?

Like my red new shoes very much. Think I'll wear them for the first time Saturday. Know you'll like them, too.

Arrive in town this evening at 4:40, exactly a 20–minute ride from the Works. "Sharpey" certainly is a speed demon—50 miles P.H. all the way in Joliet. Had plenty of time to do a little shopping, but nothing was accomplished in an hour.

Dearest, I love you very much. I don't really know what I'd do without you if anything should occur. I'd miss you terribly. I'd probably have to leave town to forget you. But that's something we won't discuss at present. Do you still love me?

How's that nasty cold of yours? I do hope it's gone. It should be if you practiced what you usually preach, that is, about my taking care of myself. Do take care of yourself. You have me worried.

All my love,

Trude

P.S. I love you very much.

In those days, mail was supposed to come twice a day, and she was lamenting no letters from me in either delivery. She wasn't above laying the guilt on rather thick in her letters as well. And she could still not resist telling me about her active social life, knowing I was trapped in my room studying.

I was so wild about her that even this craziness didn't send me fleeing.

December 16, 1942

My dearest, sweetest Trude:

I love you very much my darling and miss your "whooper-doo" kisses. Your letter was very encouraging honey, and I hope you have forgotten what you told me Sunday afternoon about our separation.

I'm glad you liked the flowers I sent to you, celebrating our 6 month anniversary. Maybe our next one will be crowned with a more valuable gift. Would it be all right with you?

Tomorrow, we have our Chem exam. Once again, I think I know the material but I'll probably have an amnesia attack and forget everything I know. Let's hope nothing like that occurs. I'll have to pray hard this evening for a little spiritual aid. It usually helps me quite a bit so, "Praise the Lord and pass the knowledge."

A rumor has been initiated around school that we might have to wear uniforms (either Buck Private or 2nd lieutenant uniforms). I hope the government decides on the latter, since the outfit worn by privates is not too smooth-looking. How do you think I'd look in a Khaki suit? Slick, huh?

Well, sweetheart it is 8 pm and I have to hit the books again. Monotonous, isn't it? Pretty soon I'll have my leave of absence for two weeks and will be free from work.

Bye for now. Be good. See you Saturday.

All my love and kisses,

Dick

P.S. Our code forever.

P.S. I love you my one and only above all things.

We were both getting excited as Christmas break approached and we would have more time to spend together. And I hoped we would have time to work out whatever her problem was once and for all.

12/17/42

Thursday, 1:00 p.m.

Dearest darling Dick,

Just returned from lunch and have a few moments to spare. So the best thing to do is write to you. Was your exam easy? It certainly is a relief having that off your chest. What a wonderful two week period you have to look forward to. Wish I could get a vacation soon. My two weeks I'm taking the last two weeks in February.

Had a fair time at the Oh Henry last night. There were exactly 18 couples present. On Saturday night they have a Wednesday night's attendance. Approximately 400 people compared with the 2,000 before gas rationing commenced. Really is fun being there when the attendance is so low. Seems like a privately owned ballroom. Can try all the new steps you desire without interference. If a party of about 5 couples went, it would really be fun. The service is excellent. Russ Carlyle played last night, and he didn't contribute much to the liveliness of the group.

Got home at 1:30 a.m. and was a fairly good girl. Was always hoping it was you instead of my last-nite friend. It didn't harm our relationship in the least. As a matter of fact, it made me appreciate you more, and I'm sure my love for you has grown immensely since last night. Maybe I ought to do it more often. What do you think?

I do hope I have at least one letter from you this evening. I certainly missed it yesterday. It is disappointing, isn't it?

Your flowers certainly do look gorgeous on the dining room table. They're still surviving. Incidentally, the orchid is still in the refrigerator. It's ready for the morgue or the encyclopedia.

Lots of love,

Trude

P.S. I love you very much.

Once again she was coyly teasing about following my wishes while still doing exactly what she wanted. But one good thing that came out of all of these trials and tribulations was that she now felt the need to reassure me of her love over and over again, which I very much appreciated.

December 17, 1942

My sweetest Trude:

The semester is just about over and I'm pretty glad that I have completed it. The final test in Chemistry wasn't too hard and I knew something about each question. If the instructors who grade the papers are lenient, I may pass. Any how, I hope I come through without flunking. The lowest grade that I can get is a 75 in order to have a C- average which in my estimation, is lousy. No doubt, when I get back January 4th they'll give me my walking papers. Woe to me if that happens.

According to the paper, we med students are being called to active duty and this will occur at the end of this academic year. The government will assume all responsibilities and we will be under their supervision. Nice, huh? What a mess this is turning out to be.

Well, Dearie, I'll be seeing you Saturday. In exactly 50 hours I'll be kissing you again. That will be the best moment of the whole week. I love you so much that I can't live without you, honey, and don't forget to "keep trying."

I guess I'll have to close now and head for the dinner table. Not much to
do tonite except read a little Anatomy. See you soon—he quicker the better.
   All my love and kisses,
   Dick
   P.S. Our code forever
   P.S. I love you, I love you, I love you, very much.
   P.S. In all my life, I have never had the pleasure of being with such a
nice considerate, pretty girl!!

We spent a wonderful first Christmas together. I went home each
night imagining what it would be like to not have to go home at a certain time; to really spend Christmas together each year for the rest of
our lives.

I returned to school missing her, but also never having been happier in my life.

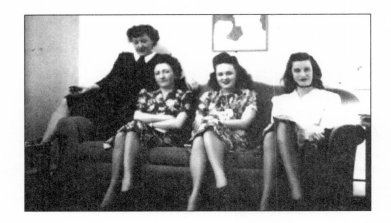

Trude (at right) with
some of her coworkers
at the Purity Baking
Company. (top)

Me as a private in the US
army

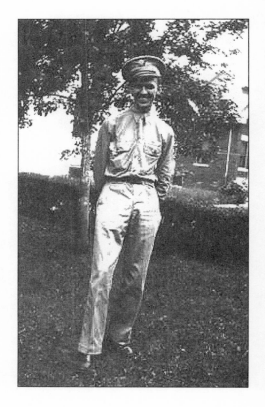

Trude and I Get Closer

We resumed writing as soon as I was back at school. I liked hearing all of the details of her work, home, and happenings back in Joliet. Once I was back at school, she had a different kind of little scare for me, but I knew it could not be too serious because of her little jokes about it:

> January 11, 1943
>
> (Monday)
>
> Dearest Darling Dick,
>
> Was almost in 7th heaven this evening. Upon our return from work, in dear Sharpe's car, Viv and I were very comfortably seated in the back seat with not a care in the world. Suddenly it seemed as if we were on the Tilt-a-Whirl, or the Boomerang. I don't know what Sharpe was trying to do, but I do know what the car was doing. The road was pretty slick, the car spun around, and we landed in the ditch. Headed in the opposite direction. Luckily, there were no cars too close or we would have crashed. Viv and I were saying our prayers and I'm not kidding. It certainly was a breath-taking experience. To top it all, Sharpe had trouble getting out of the ditch and me anticipating to make the 5 o'clock bus for Chicago. (I didn't, took the 5:30.) "You'd be so nice to come home to" is now being played by Chico Marx's Orch. Whose song? Viv and I decided to help by getting out of the car and pushing. Stopped in snow knee-deep & the spinning wheels of the car dug down into the wet snow & splattered us with the clean black mud. At that point, I decided to quit & went out on the road and "hitched" a ride. Had no trouble getting one due to the great amount of traffic. 3 cars stopped

& we arrived in town at 5:00 pm, too late to get the 5 o'clock bus. Did get to Chicago nevertheless.

Ethel spoke very highly of you today. I guess you made a "hit" with her. (as you do with all women) She thinks you are very nice. Of course, I do too and then some.

It's getting rather late, 11:30 pm. Dearest, I love you very much. Miss you so much that I'm counting the hours and days till I see you again. Think of you constantly. You're probably in the midst of one of your lessons at this time. Do take it easy. & don't work yourself into a frazzle. Please consider your health for there is the future to think of. Agreed? Goodbye for now.

All my love, always

Trude

P.S. I love you very much, steady.

She was doing a wonderful job keeping up her daily letters which always brightened my days.

1/12/43

Tuesday

Dearest darling Steady,

Your two very sweet letters were received & read with much pleasure & delight. I do think that Saturday was the most perfect & wonderful evening we've spent in some time. It should, & will be, no doubt, a memorable evening, for on that decisive day, the futures of 2 people that were at stake were decided upon. Am very happy that we are still "steadying" it. The few years will pass quickly & we'll be together for always. I know we'll get along beautifully. What is your opinion?

Think I'll go to the movies tomorrow nite. Crossroads is playing at the Mode & the Ink Spots are at the Rialto. Will have to hold someone else's hand, though. This I won't enjoy too much.

One of the girls at DuPonts saw "The Eve of St. Mark," said it was very good & thought we'd enjoy it.

Darling I do love you very much and often wonder I am doing the right thing. But I guess I thought about it long enough to know. You're very sweet to forgive sincerely something you don't even know. You'll always rank "tops" with me, sweetie. Truthfully, I do not think anyone can compare with you. Miss you very much. Will see you Saturday. You'll call me if you have time, won't you? Goodbye for now.

All my love,

Trude

I still was wondering what she had done. But I also knew I was not likely to ever find out, so there was not much point in asking any more. So in my reply, after reacting to the frightening story of her mishap, I decided to try my hand at a love poem:

January 14, 1943

My dearest Trude,

Today, I had my exam in Psychiatry. Boy, was it a joke. There were 5 definitions and a choice of 2 essay questions. To think I studied for 2 nights for such a course is most annoying. If I had the slightest inclination that the material was to be so compact, I wouldn't have opened a sheet of the syllabus. Medical School is sure tough!!

I read your letter with my heart in my mouth. When I read of your hair-raising experience, I was all set to say a prayer that Sharpe would learn to drive. I do wish he would take more care when he's taking you home. After all I don't want to hear that you have been in an accident or something like that. Inform him that he better give more heed to the welfare of my future wife. Or else, I'll have to reprimand him when I get home on Saturday.

Well, darling, today is Wednesday and I think I have been gone a year already. I love you so very much that when I look at your picture, I feel as if I have the world right where I want it. Gee, you're pretty—as my roommates have mentioned also, numerous times. They want to meet you so they can get a look at a smooth girl. I'll give them a chance at our formal—if they're good to me till then.

How do you like it? Out of my own little head:

"A girl named Trude cannot be beat

She's nice and pretty and oh, so sweet,

I tell her I love her, would be no lie,

For her alone, would I want to die."

All my love & kisses,

Dick

P.S. Our codes forever.

She appreciated my poor attempt at poetry and wrote to me about it, but then gave me yet another scare of a different kind.

1/14/43

Thursday

Dearest darling,

Your poetic ability really astonished me. Don't know why I was so amazed, for I should have known you were capable of almost anything. It was a very beautiful poem, & have been thinking of starting a collection. Good idea?

Ethel asked me again today if we would like to double with them Saturday. I told them I'd ask you if you had already made plans. I suppose it would be fun to have chaperones. What do you think?

A "Good Neighbor Car-Sharing Drive" will commence next Monday. Dad is Zone Chief for the N.E. Zone & his Civilian Defense workers had their meeting in the Funeral Home this evening at 7:00. Fancy that.

(Had another brainstorm. Have been thinking quite seriously of enlisting in the Waves. Sounds quite promising. The duties of a Wave take place only in the U.S. Occupations include office work, radio operator, meteorologists, aerologists, air traffic controllers, link trainer operators & parachute maintenance workers. The last isn't at all appealing; next to last, I don't even know what that is.

The work I'd like best is the one requiring the most training. No office work for me. The drive for recruits is open until Sat. night. The only thing holding me up is the approval of 3 people—Mom-Dad-you. Might not be too difficult to obtain since a Wave's duties take place only in the U.S. Here's hoping. I have my fingers crossed. It would be an interesting experience & a patriotic gesture, don't you think so, since there is a great need for Waves? DuPont's would have to release me then.)

Sweetheart, I think I'll bid you adieu. I don't feel very well. The day
was miserable. It seems that I'm always ailing. How is your health these
days?

My love for you has grown
Since the days and weeks have flown.
But our big day, Saturday, is near
And I'm really looking forward to it, dear.
How's that?

[She then filled half a page with shorthand squiggles.]

I'm sorry to keep you in the dark in regard to the above. The hieroglyph-
ics are only my shorthand notes for "Please think of me." Bing Crosby just
completed singing the song. Another one of my songs. Miss you terribly,
love. Love you very much. Think of you always, love.

All my love, forever,
Trude

P.S. I love you, our codes forever.
2 P.S. Happy anniversary, dear! I noted that you confused your dates.
Yesterday's letter was dated the 14th. Just a speedy kid, Dick. Think I'll get
you a calendar. A discrepancy in your dates might prove disastrous.

Sometimes I wondered how serious she was about some of these
ideas, or did she just throw them out to drive me crazy? I know she
desperately wanted out of that cramped little house and out of Joliet
and joining the women's branch of the Navy could be her ticket to
see the world, or, at least, another part of the country. As essential
defense work, DuPont could make it difficult for employees to leave.
Trude's mother, father and I all disapproved of her joining the Waves,
so she let it drop for the time being, but it was not the last time she
raised that possibility.

January 14, 1943
My dearest Trude,

In about a half an hour, I have to play basketball with the house. Little
relaxation after a hard exam. Ha! Ha! I'll probably be exhausted after the
night of exercise. First time in about 2 months.

Your letter was terrific. It sure gives me a lift in the heart to read such a wonderful masterpiece. Talking about sweet letters, yours is tops. I'm glad you think the years will pass quickly because I hope the same. The faster the better for me.

Concerning your gazing at rings, I think that Lebolt's display is magnificent also. I've seen it a few times when I was downtown and there are some beautiful stones in the display. Not too expensive, either. Only $1000 or 2. Drop in the bucket for wealthy people. Right?

Sweetheart, I love you immensely and I treasure you above everything else in the world. Will you marry me? (I'm proposing) That's swell. I think of you of being with you most of the time and I dream of you every night. In other words, I LOVE YOU VERY MUCH!

Goodbye for tonight. Think of you often and I'll see you Saturday. Will call when I get in.

All of my love & kisses,

Dick

P.S. Our code forever and ever.

"With you I'll spend all of my life
I know you'll be the very best wife.
Nothing on earth can take your place
Before me always will be your face."

At some point we had both started assuming we would get married. I'm not sure when that assumption took hold, but the fact that we were both looking at wedding rings so soon after our threatened separation meant we must have resolved it very well. I decided I wanted to formalize our relationship. I had been wanting that for a long time, perhaps since I first saw her photo in the paper. But Trude was still not ready to commit, or at least wanted to wait until I finished school.

1/20/43

Thursday

Hello again sweetie,

Just finished reading your letters. They're so sweet that I sit reading them with the brightest smile.

I miss you very much & am wondering how you are bearing these sub-zero temperatures. 20 below here this morning was really an experience. Don't believe I've ever been out at a time that it was as cold as today. Arrived at work late today—36 minutes to be exact. Sharp was a bit leery about taking out his car. So—we had an early start on the bus from home, 20 after 6. Arrived in town at 6:30, at which time the first bus left for duPonts. We weren't able to take it—overcrowded. Waited for the 6:40 which didn't show up, likewise, for the 6:50 and 7:00. Sharp gave up and decided to go home for his car. In the meantime, we were having loads of fun in the bus depot with the men from Central Shops. They were a very congenial group. We weren't at all anxious to get out to the Plant, but Mr. Sharp has a family to support & every dollar counts. He came up at 7:45 & we were on our merry way, arriving at the time clock at 8:21. Everyone was at work except George. He's still snowbound.

Dearest, I do think you might measure up to the qualifications of a very good & later a famous poet. Perhaps you should give it more serious thought. Take it from a world-renowned critic. (It slipped, that's a bit too strong.)

You write of making the time we need be apart shorter. Sweetie, I don't know what you mean. I know five years is a long time, but the obstacles causing this long separation are so great that it is impossible to do anything about it. You know that I feel as you do & would do anything to hasten matters.

Yes, the day after celebrating my birthday, I'll celebrate our 8th month anniversary. Do you know that you first wrote me on March 13, making it almost a year. Significant dates: 13th of March—your first letter to me, 13th of February—my birthday; a difference of one month, the important date being a month after my birthday. 14th of June, our going steady, 14th of July—your birthday a difference of one month, the important date being a month before your birthday. Coincidence, isn't it? Wonder if it's good or bad luck? I'll be optimistic and say it's good, no doubt about it.

Sweetheart, I dream of you most of the day & it feels very good. It seems to soothe my loneliness for you. It's terrible to feel lonely, don't you

think? But ours does have a compensation—weekends. All people aren't as
fortunate as we. Aren't we lucky? Don't forget your plans of greeting when
you arrive for our date promptly next Saturday. I'm so sorry to have been so
provoked last Saturday, but waiting for you I had time to think & thought if
you really loved me & missed me so terribly, you'd at least be on time for our
weekly dates. Do you understand now? I don't know if I explained this
before, but I was quite disappointed which made me very obstinate. So very
sorry.

 I love you so much, Dick, that I'd like to sit & write to you all day long.
I do think of you so much. Only 3 more days & I'll see you again. Till then
I'll eagerly be awaiting your return.

 All my love, always,
 Trude
 P.S. Our code forever.

[then a few more lines of Gregg squiggles.]

 Decoded:

 I love you very much, sweetheart. Miss you so terribly that I don't know
what I'll do without you. Please stay well and healthy for my sake, sweetie.

 2 P.S. If we keep this up, either you'll learn shorthand or I'll learn
German.

She had the sweetest way of keeping me on my toes and reprimanding me for being late, but still she made it clear she was out having a good time now and then. Her being upset at me for being late
made me appreciate how she valued our limited time together and
she felt cheated that I had deprived her of even one minute of it. Her
life was pretty mundane and my weekly visits made both of our lives
more bearable.

 February 4, 1943
 7:35 a.m.
 Dearest Darling,

 Good morning, dear. Sorry I'm late in writing, but I arrived home
rather late from Ethel's party—2:00 a.m. We all had a grand time & the
dinner was super. We played pinocle (I think that's spelled correctly?) &
now I believe I can play with all the pros at your frat house and beat them

*too. Maybe you and I ought to play sometime. Think it's loads of fun. And
don't forget about teaching me to play bridge.*

*Didn't receive a letter yesterday. Believe it is the fault of the U.S. Post
Office, and not yours. Was a little disappointed, for I expected one to read
upon my return from the party.*

*One of Ethel's boyfriends accommodated me with a ride home. He was-
n't a gentleman at all because he wouldn't take me to the door. It was very
dark, too. He ask me if I went to the dance Ethel attended, but I just said
'no.' I didn't tell him I was going steady. Should I have? He was very nice,
but he certainly did not compare with you, sweetheart, my one and only.*

*Goodbye for now, sweetie. The engineers are telling me that I'm at work
now & I certainly can take a hint.*

All my love, always

Trude

She then ended this letter with a kiss—a lipstick imprint of her lips.
Such little touches would drive me wild, and I would have a hard time
thinking of anything but her soft warm lips until the next time we
met. I kept pressing for more, but she would deal with my surging
emotions by telling me about someone watching from above, and
consoling me that some day, not too far in the future, we'd always be
together. That usually helped cool my engines a little, but with each
caress I found it more and more difficult to restrain my young emotions. After all, what was I to do when I would press my body to hers
and feel her breasts against me? It was almost more than a healthy
young man could resist. But of course in those days, premarital sex
was almost unheard of, and good girls like Trude would never let
themselves be pressured into going farther than they should with a
guy.

February 9, 1943

Tuesday evening

My one and only forever,

*Good evening my darling. Received your letter this morning and I
enjoyed it very much. Sorry to hear you were so tired Sunday evening. I
hope I didn't cause your feeling the way you did. I felt a little tired Sunday*

also, but I don't think it was due to actual fatigue but just being blue and feeling so lonely up here without you.

Tomorrow is the day of reckoning. I pray that my brains are in working order so I can really hit this test. Your prayers last Friday & Saturday will aid me terrifically, I know. They did last time—I'm sure I'll have the same success tomorrow.

Joe. L. called this evening and notified me that he can't make it Saturday. He's low on funds and thinks he had better wait till a further date to go along with us. If you want to go, we can still make it, but what you think, is what we shall do.

Would you like to go to the Northwestern-Illinois basketball game Feb. 27th? We haven't seen one this year. Would be fun don't you think? Tell me what you decide.

Some of the fellows from the house are going, including Sauer and Kirchhoff, and maybe a party afterwards will ensue—not a "brawl" though.

Dearest darling, I love you very, very much—more and more every day. Gee, I wish we could get married then we would be together always. I miss you so much that my heart pines for you day and night and to be with you is my wish all the time we are apart. Be good sweetheart. Take care of yourself (I wear my boots every day—it's pretty wet up here.)

All my love and kisses

Dick

P.S. Our codes forever and ever

P.S. "Good nite little angel"

P.S. Happy Birthday, dearest one.

Once again I got my days and dates mixed up since the 9th could not have been a Tuesday and the 10th a Thursday. I also filled my letters with the mundane details of my life, but somehow they never seemed as interesting as hers.

February 10, 1943

My sweetest Trude,

Love is swell, isn't it, honey? As I said Sunday, I don't think there are two persons as much in love as we are. I suppose everybody in town knows that anyhow, but maybe we should publish it to the world and give other people a few instructions, right?

I do hope you get your raise very soon. I imagine it would come in handy if you could get it before your vacation commences. Where do you intend to go when your vacation starts? You haven't told me as yet. Hope you don't go away because I'll miss you terribly if I couldn't see you every weekend and receive your weekly supply of letters.

I have one more test to take. It is in Pharmacology and I would like to get a good grade in it. Thus far this week, I haven't done too well. The more we recapitulate among ourselves, the grades drop 10 points. Seems as if I am getting dumber day by day. I can't figure it out. You know how hard I study, cause I do so much want to be a great doctor-husband for you and to be just a quack is worthless. I think I had better find some brain cells somewhere.

Bye for now. Love you and you are "Always in my heart."

All my love & kisses

Dick

P.S. Our codes forever & ever. xxx

2P.S. I wish that I could write shorthand. xxx

Then we could both write in the same way. xxx

Of course we had our little disagreements, as when she sarcastically took me to task for canceling plans without consulting her and then again threatened to join the service, so it made me wonder all the more if these supposed plans of hers were really just a way of keeping me in line:

2/10/43

Wednesday

Hi Hon,

I'm very disappointed to hear that our plans for Saturday evening have fallen through. You say, "if you (me) want to go, we can still make it." Evidently I didn't convince you, or bring it across to you, that I really wanted to see the play Saturday. Of course, if you don't think that would be wise, or so much fun to go alone, all well & good. Anything you say, you

seem to be the boss. Perhaps we can go some other time. Why not make it a
surprise so that another plan doesn't fail.

In regard to the Ill-N.W. game Feb 27, I won't count on going. So many
things seem to happen in a week's or 2 weeks' time that I foresee these plans fail-
ing also. I'm getting tired of looking forward to exciting weekends and having
plans changed when the anticipated event is at hand. Perhaps I'm wrong in
thinking or feeling as I do. What do you think? Please don't let anything written
thus far upset you. Frankly, that is how I feel about our plans, at present.

Hope you've finished your 4 or 5 exams. I remember you in all my
prayers & hope you make the grade in all your dreaded Xams. Incidentally,
how were the exams you already had?

Glad to hear that you're wearing your boots. I am also. It's quite wet &
muddy on the Works, but by tomorrow, no doubt I'll be walking thru snow.
It's getting quite cold outdoors. Noticed this while walking home from shop-
ping this evening. Missed both buses.

Had another brainstorm about enlisting in the Waves. This time I'll do
less talking & more acting. I erred the last time in telling everyone, for they
just talked me out of it. Elaine's thinking of the Waacs. I wonder who'll
act first.

Dearest, I love you very, very much more than anything else on earth.
My one wish is to be with you for always & always. After 5 years this wish
will be fulfilled. By then this horrible war should be ended (I hope) and I'll
be back from the Waves. Then I can tell you in detail all of my experiences in
the service, while sitting side by side in our living room before the fireplace
(might have to be imaginary). My, that is a beautiful thought, isn't it, dear?

Goodnight, my love. Will be thinking of you until I see you again.

All my love forever, always

Trude

P.S. I love you.

Once again she threatened to join the Women's branch of the
Navy, which after her rebukes did seem more of an idle threat than a
real plan. After she was done scolding me, she told me how much she
loved me, so I was a little relieved, but the chastisement continued
into her next letter.

February 11, 1943

Dearest Dick,

I'm feeling neglected this week. To date I've received 2 letters, usually I have 4. Perhaps with your 4 exams this week, you've had no time to write to me. Or, the mail service isn't as efficient as usual. Don't know what to think of it but it will make easier what I plan to do in the very near future. Will tell you about it Saturday. It's nothing to get alarmed about.

While writing my Thursday nite letters to you, I keep thinking that Saturday evenings, when I can see you again are very near. In reality, they're not; for I have exactly 48 hours to wait before our weekly date—and that's really a long time for a couple in love as much as we are. Right? Our many short separations will soon be eliminated won't they? (5 yrs). Do you think a long separation would be a wise replacement?

You probably feel relieved to have your exams completed. Hope you did well & ranked in the very top bracket of your class. Know you did, for you're just a "genius."

Met an old friend on the bus this evening. She joined the Waac's & was just returning from Chicago where she spent the last 2 days at the government's expense, taking physical & mental tests. She was very fortunate in passing both, for only one out of every two were fortunate to pass both exams. She expects to leave in about 20 days. Lucky girl!! Now I'm more serious than ever about joining the Waves. Wish me luck dearest. I know I'll like it.

In just 2 days I won't be as lonely as I am this evening. I'll be seeing you again and will be loving you as much as ever. It feels very good to see you dearest, and I hope the time won't pass too slowly.

Goodnight, one and only, forever. Will see you soon & hope that I have a better tomorrow. If not, I'll know something is wrong.

All my love, always

Trude

P.S. I love you very, very, very much always.

In our talks and dates, we always seemed to patch things up nicely. She could be coy and made sure I kept up the chase and never took anything, including our Saturday night dates, for granted.

February 16, 1943

Dearest Dick,

Am listening to "Famous Jury Trials." The story involves a young medical student. Half the things I read or hear bring thoughts of you. Another reminder is the novel I'm reading, "Hostess of the Skyways." One of the characters is a Mr. Zoller & every time I see the name I think of you. Very enjoyable, pleasant thoughts.

Am looking forward to my vacation coming up next week. Intend to take it very easy and rest as much as possible. Too bad you don't have a vacation, also. If you did, we'd be able to see each other daily. Wouldn't that be super? Will no doubt be in Chicago next week. Can at least buzz you sweetie.

I'm so very glad that we have definitely come to an understanding about different important things. Let's live up to our promise or resolutions or what have you. I feel so relieved that we talked things over. I've really been giving it a great deal of thought. Now, my mind is at ease and at peace with the One that really counts. How about you? Of course, I know it's a delicate subject but we needn't worry about that any longer. Let's start over again from the beginning & make things right. I hope it doesn't trouble you too much. Let's forget it ever occurred. That's that.

Sweetie, I love you very much and I hope you didn't believe me when I said I didn't care to go out with you Saturday nite. Of course, I sounded very convincing I know, but I can put acts on when I want to. I'd rather be with you than anyone else on earth and if you thought I really intended to break our date, and go with Viv to some old dance & dance all nite with a lot of jerks & dulls (as you'd call them) I guess you still don't really know or understand me. As long as I love you as much as I do, and you should know I couldn't fall out of love in one night, and that if I didn't love you any more I'd say so, instead of leading you on. I'll never, never break any date with you. After all, it seems as though we're together so short a time, and to break a date, especially on a Saturday nite would simply be out of the question, and positively the improper thing to do. What do you think? I miss you more than I can ever convey in speech or writing. I would like to be with you, my one and only sweetheart every day & every nite until the end of time. Please believe me. And get all those foolish ideas about my thinking of breaking up

*out of your head, Dearest. It's 11:20 & I think Ill drift into dreamland &
keep our all important date. What date? Our wedding date. I can dream,
can't I?*

*To date haven't heard from you. Course, I didn't expect to. Will be look-
ing for your "sugar report" tomorrow. Until then, I'll be thinking of you.
Good-nite Dick. Will see you in my dreams.*

All my love, forever.

Trude.

P.S. I love you very much, always and always

She always kept dangling our future wedding in front of me like the
carrot just out of reach by warding off my advancing and promising
me "soon," and at the same time telling me it was years away. By the
spring of 1943, we were both getting tired of the long-distance
romance, and she was tired of the lengthy and sometimes perilous
commute to DuPont down in Elwood, so she started looking for a job
in Chicago. Once again she had given up (at least for the moment)
her idea about joining the Waves. In April, she gave her notice after
being hired as executive secretary to a vice-president at the Purity
Baking Company. The pay was the same, $100 a week, but it would
be for working five days instead of the five and a half required at the
ordnance plant.

The office manager at the defense plant asked her to stay on when
he learned of her plans, but Trude had made up her mind to leave.
Commuter-rail service between Joliet and Chicago was quite depend-
able, but she also immediately started looking for a place to live in the
city. She found a place at the Franciscan Girl's Club—a rooming
house on Michigan Avenue where she shared a room with another
girl, Dorothy. Now she was only a trolley ride away from me.

Often, after my evening meal I'd hop on the Paulina Street trolley.
There was a stop just a few steps from where I lived, and within 20
minutes I'd be at Chicago and State Street on the north side of the
city. I'd spend a few delightful hours with Trude, and then head back
home to my lodgings at the Nu Sigma Nu house. One other wonderful advantage of her being in the city was that she was now a nickel

phone call away, although getting the phone or privacy in the frat house or her rooming house wasn't always easy.

We still couldn't see each other every day, although we saw each other much more often. The letters helped us spend time with each other every day. Her letter of April 13 included a nice P.S., and it was things like this that kept me on edge through our entire courtship.

> *P.S. I love you more and more each day. Can it be possible to love one as much as I love you and you love me? Think we will be able to wait three whole years for the great and eventful day? We must I know but the question is how are we going to do it? Something will have be done and very soon. What do you suggest? I still cannot understand how it occurred so quickly. It is just ten months you know. It is wonderful and I am very glad and happy and I am hoping that the three years pass quickly.*

> *Flash! Just had an idea. Perhaps we could sleep off a few years: our problem would be solved, but what about your schooling? No, that wouldn't work for you. Darn it! (I know what we can do—just wait) Why didn't we think of that before? No more worries for a while now that we have that solved.*

We went on writing back and forth. One letter she wrote in April was entirely in shorthand and I had to eagerly wait for her to translate it. Whether in shorthand or her neat script, she always gushed with an enthusiasm about even the smallest details of her life that let me know her better, had me wanting to know her more, and provided a welcome break from my studies.

> *7:30 a.m.*

> *4/15/43*

> *My dearest darling,*

> *Had a great time last evening dearest. Our 10–month anniversary was lots of fun, and I've been thinking that no doubt our 10th year anniversary will be celebrated going to the show and drinking grape rickeys. I was sorry to see you leave so soon, but since our time is not our own actually, we do have to abide by certain rules. Right?*

> *I hope you got to bed shortly after 12:00 and did not do any studying. You're a mastermind anyway and you needn't study too much. It's wonderful to have a photographic mind, isn't it? Will say those prayers for you*

tonight so that you would make a very good grade in your exams tomorrow. You can count on me. I wouldn't worry about them if I were you, though.

Thank Kirk for me for trying to get an invite to the K.D. dance Saturday nite. It was very thoughtful and nice of him. It would be fun, but to the show in Joliet with you is fun, too. Think I'll have to scoot now. It's almost 7:40 and I still have to get some breakfast before 8:00. Will be thinking of you, as I always do. Don't work too hard. Will call tonight.

Remember that I love you very much, and will for always & always. You're my one and only, you know, and to be with you and yours forever is one of my favorite dreams.

Goodbye for now, sweetheart.

All my love & kisses,

Trude

P.S. Our codes forever & ever & ever.

I love you, I love you, I love you, always will. Miss you terribly. Think of you always.

She filled me with the details of her life and since she no longer had her sisters in which to confide, she would tell me everything that was going on with her. It made me feel closer on those nights when we could not be together.

Tuesday, April 27

Dearest Darling, One & Only,

Just completed an 8-page letter to Elaine. Told Elaine about our wonderful dates and plans for next weekend. Had a grand time reviewing our dates. We certainly have been doing a variety of things. It was wonderful, dearest, & I enjoyed every minute of it. The next weekend I'm sure will be very very very enjoyable. Can't wait.

Am listening to your radio & it isn't acting up at all tonite. Bob Hope's program is on now & Jerry Colonna is singing. He's very good.

My roommate just finished ironing and is awfully thirsty for a coke. She's always wanting something & too lazy to go out for it. Poor girl. Wish you were here instead. Incidentally, don't forget that sweater you want me to wash for you.

Ours must be one of the greatest and truest loves in history. What do you think? Romeo's & Juliet's is very mild compared with ours. Right? I think it's super—super to love each other as we do. It makes life interesting and takes the dullness out of it. Agreed? Really, I don't know what we'd do without each other. We'd probably feel lifeless and blue and sad and would probably shrivel up and be blown away by the wind. (Wonderful imagination, don't you think?)

Goodnite, loved one. Will see you tomorrow nite. Will be thinking of you & loving you very much.

All my love & kisses,

Trude

P.S. Our codes forever & ever.

I love you, I miss you, I think of you always. Ditto, ditto, ditto.

XXXXX = 5 big whopperdoos that you can collect tomorrow.

We often closed our letters with "xxxx" for kisses or sometimes she would use "888" for hugs, a code she said she learned from some Navy guys she and Viv met in Chicago. What she was doing receiving even written hugs from a sailor, I didn't want to ask. I knew she wrote to some friends and relatives in the service, and most girls felt it was their patriotic duty to make sure the boys off fighting the war got some mail from home, but often it worried me as to what she was writing to whom.

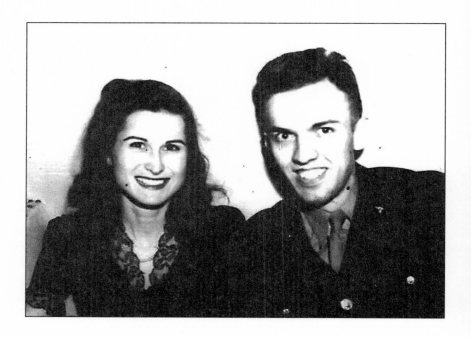

Me with Trude after I
was in uniform. (top)

Trude and me (at right)
with some friends at
the beach in Chicago.

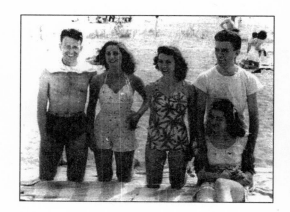

Closing in on the Ring

On carrousels in those days there was often a brass ring on a hook, and if you could catch it as your horse rode by, you could redeem that ring for a free ride or some other prize. At times I felt like I was on a merry-go-round of Trude's making. She had me up and she had me down and running in circles, but most of the time there was fun music playing as I laughed and enjoyed myself just being with her or thinking of her. Instead of me reaching out to grab the ring, however, I was holding out an engagement ring and hoping that one of these times she would grab it. She had many legitimate reasons to not want to marry me just yet, not the least of which was I had no money and she wasn't making enough to support us both.

There were other obstacles as well, including how hard it might be for me to get any studying done if I had to share a small apartment with such a lovely distraction. I was willing to take that chance, but overcoming the cash problem was a little more difficult until the Army came to my rescue.

Along with 20,000 other medical students, I was about to become an active member of the military. The reserve status in which I had remained since registering for the draft in 1941 changed and I was about to put on a uniform. Unfortunately, we were made privates instead of officers, so the uniform and pay were not as nice as I had hoped. The good news was that Uncle Sam would now pay my tuition and expenses, and I'd be making army pay just for going to school. I would now be self-sufficient, which eliminated one of Trude's excuses for us not getting married immediately.

My fellow medical students and I would now belong to the Army and were put on an accelerated program with all unnecessary classes eliminated. We would go straight through with no breaks to complete our studies in the shortest time possible. It added a lot of stress, as though medical school wasn't tough enough—and I wasn't the smartest person in my class of 186 students.

While many of my classmates saw our being called to active duty as a calamity—we were no longer free to choose our futures—I accepted it in stride.

I planned to use this to try to talk Trude into an earlier wedding date, and as time went on, I was wearing her down. She went from talking about five years to three years.

Monday

April, May 3, 1943

My darling,

Excuse the misdated heading, but I'm still in a daze after our wonderful evening together. Did you have a good time my love? I hope I kept all of my promises—the ones agreed to last week. I didn't break them, did I? I'm sure you will agree that I was a good boy, right?

You are so sweet, Trude, that 3 years will be like eternity. Wish you could condescend to marry me after I get into the Army in July. Just think $130 a month and I could spend all of it on you. I would enjoy that very, very much my love if you would permit me. Will you think about it seriously? Please, honey.

Will be waiting anxiously to see you Wed. evening. We won't be able to stay out too late but to see you for just a few minutes, when I miss you so much is wonderful

I just got home a little late last night , but I'm not too tired today. Dreamed of you last evening. You were swimming with another girl at the Nowell pool and I happened to be there also—don't know how I got there, though. As soon as I saw you, I dove into the water and when you noticed me you went underwater to see if I could find you. It seemed I looked around for hours but no sign of Trude. When I finally came to the surface, who was sitting on the wall, but you—grinning from ear to ear. But then I

caught you and pulled you in and the last thing I remember you were in my
arms and I was in heaven, I know. Pretty nice, huh?

Have to start grinding now, sweetie and will await your call eagerly.
Don't work too hard and think of me when you have some free time.
Goodnite my one and only forever. I love you, I love you, immensely, terrifi-
cally, and just a whole lot. xxxxxxxxxxxxxxxxxxxxxxxxxxxxxxxxxx.

All my love & kisses,

Dick

P.S. Our codes forever & ever & ever.

She responded to my suggestion with enthusiasm, if not a firm yes
and a wedding date.

Dearest Darling,

Good morning my one & only, my first thoughts, as usual, are of you. I
missed you lots last nite, more after our telephone conversation. Thought it
was very nice and certainly out of the ordinary.

I've been thinking about your question very seriously and will give it
more thought, of course. I think it would be super to do as you ask, it cer-
tainly would solve many things. Whee!!! Being together for always &
always. It makes me feel very good. Am anxious to see your letter, even
though I know what it is all about. It will make me feel heavenly again to
see it in writing after hearing it. Ever since last evening, time—10:30, I've
been singing & humming "I'm in love with you, honey." Can't get the song
out of my mind, of course, I don't want to.

Was surprised last evening when I arrived home. Dorothy had finally
found that much talked-about and sought for apartment where she can
cook. It accommodates one & is very small, but it is what she wants &
she is moving out today. I'm sorry to see her go, for I thought she was
very nice & we were just getting to know each other. I'll miss her iron,
too. Now I'll have to hunt until I find one, if that's possible. Wish me
luck.

I'll have to go now. Goodbye for now. I'll be anxiously awaiting your
call this evening. Think of me & don't work too hard.

All my love & kisses, always,

Trude

ETA of Nu Sigma Nu
626 S. Ashland Blvd
Chicago, Illinois
May 4, 1943
Dearest sweetheart Trude:

I feel wonderful after our telephone conversation last evening. It was very enjoyable and I hope that you will think of my proposal. Wouldn't it be nice if you and I could get married sooner than expected? I would be very, very happy if you would consent.

I love you my darling very, very, very, very much. You are to me every-thing—and you will be my one and only forever. I send thousands of kisses to you and each one is from the bottom of my heart. Can I continue to kiss you as many times as I want? I hope so, cause you are so nice to hold and kiss and every time your lips touch mine—you know what happens. Ah, love is wonderful. Isn't it, lovely one?

I almost forgot to tell you I received a letter from Whitey Bergstrom—remember him? He's aboard the S.S. San Diego somewhere in the South Seas. He's having quite a time according to the contents of the letter but he wishes he was home. Hope he returns to dear old Joliet safely. Goodnight my love. Don't work too hard and I love you more than words can tell.

Will see you Wednesday evening. Bye
All my love & kisses,

Dick

P.S. Our codes forever & ever.
P.S. xxxx   can I
    xxxx   collect on
    xxxx   these?
    xxxx   Can't wait, my darling.

I tried to stay in touch with my friends who, one by one, were sign-ing up or being drafted. I still felt fortunate that I wasn't in combat like so many of our friends and relatives. My future brother-in-law Jack Phalen was on bombing runs over Europe. My friend Joe Limacher joined the Navy. Trude's brother Matt, Jr. ended up in the Army Air

Corps loading munitions on bombers in Burma, India, and eventually on Tinian. At one point he asked Trude for a loan to buy his girlfriend Sonia, an engagement ring. It made things a little tight for Trude on the $119.00 a month salary, but she did it even though she also had to give part of her earnings to her mother each month.

It was not hard for anyone in our age group to appreciate what going to war could mean. Many were never coming back, but none thought of those consequences, hoping against hope the bullet would travel elsewhere. A few of my pals were not so lucky. One high school classmate, Deanne Erickson, was killed early in the war when his fighter plane was hit by enemy gunfire and went down in the Pacific. Johnny Suhadolc had played first base on our team in the Nicholson Street neighborhood in Joliet. He was only 19 when he died at Anzio, never having made it off the beach-head.

The war was teaching us that life was rather precarious these days, which in my mind meant one more reason Trude and I should not wait to consummate our relationship. But I knew that could not happen until after we were married, and she was still not willing to set a date.

Often we had to force ourselves to try to put the war out of our minds and just focus on work and each other. There was so little we could do about the war for now, so for the most part we avoided it in our letters. Our letters were the bright spot in each other's days, and if there was bad news about who had been drafted or lost, we broke that in person.

Instead of her usual neat handwriting, she typed one letter to me:

May 12, 1943

10:45 a.m.

Dearest Dick,

The work in the office has let up a bit so I decided to send you a copy of the neat and good looking work I do for the people here in the office. Incidentally, I'm writing this on a piece of paper that I had wasted the other day, and that isn't speaking too well of my efficiency. We all have our off moments and days, as you undoubtedly know.

It's so beautiful outdoors that I hate staying indoors. You'll be out all afternoon enjoying the fresh spring air and sunshine. I envy you; think I'll feign illness and spend the afternoon with you. Good idea, don't you think?

Do hope we can see each other this evening for a little while. I haven't seen you since Sunday and it seems as though it has been a month. I've spent two days in—Monday and Tuesday—and had 8 hours rest each evening so I'm raring to go out and stay out until a late morning hour. Of course, that can't be done because you probably didn't receive your rest and need it badly.

Can't wait to hear of the surprise you have for me Thursday. I'm just dying of suspense. More so now than ever, because one of the girls wrote to her husband and for the past week she's been telling him that she has a surprise for him and I'll bet he's as anxious as I. He says that Sybil doesn't know the difference between a surprise and a shock, and he's certain it will turn out to be a shock. (Interesting, isn't it?)

I received a picture of our bowling team, and it is a "lu-lu" (Phil Harris). I'll bring the picture along tonight and you can see some of the people I work with.

Do hope you made the grade, sweetheart, and fooled those old army health examiners. A little wrongdoing once in a while shouldn't hurt anyone. Right? Already I can see you in that handsome private uniform. (Sigh) (Sigh) Won't you look just super. Oh boy. And won't you be proud? Did you say the boys will be in uniform the first of July? Just after our first anniversary and before your birthday. What shall we do to celebrate the three occasions? Shall we celebrate them individually in a less elaborate manner? (Don't mind me, I'm just having beautiful dreams.)

One of the girls in the office asked me yesterday if I was going steady. She was going to ask me to double with her, with one of her friend's pals, on Saturday nite. I disappointed her when I said I was going steady. My would-have-been-date is a midshipman at Abbott Hall, and according to Maybelle, very nice. Of course, he just can't compare with you, dearest, for you, in my opinion, out-shine them all. Right? That's just how I feel.

I'll be alone this evening for my roommate is going out. I don't know if I like her as much as I did in the beginning. She's very irritable but I'll have to put up with her if I want to use an iron. After I get one I might decide to move. I would like to live at the Fifth Avenue Club. Think I'll stop in and inquire about a room. If it appeals to me, I'm going to move the first opportunity I get. Then I won't have to put up with all those horrible cooking odors and interruptions by the Schmidts; and you probably won't have as much trouble getting me when you call in the evening. Will tell you more about it later.

Goodbye for now, sweetie. Will see you tonight maybe, I hope. Will be thinking of you every minute and hoping that the years standing between our important event will pass very rapidly. I do love you very much and miss you terribly.

All my love & kisses always,

Trude

P.S. Our codes forever & ever.

The Phil Harris to whom she referred was a radio comedian and bandleader who was famous for some quirky little expressions which often found their way into our everyday lives. She was concerned, as was I, that my eyesight would be rated so poor as to disqualify me from military service entirely. I passed the physical and was ready to put on a uniform. In a way, I was glad to do it. Sometimes my other friends and I got disparaging looks from the men who were in the service. Civilian status was becoming a rare commodity for men under 30, and I now felt like a member of the club instead of an outsider.

Sometimes we would go home to Joliet on weekends to see our old friends and double with Russ.

May 20, 1943

Dearest darling Dick,

About Saturday and the Oh Henry (maybe), Russ said that he'd get the gas if you got the Buick. That means that you'll drive all the way back. Don't you hate the front seat? I do. We could have so much more fun in the back. It's a half hour's ride, too. Darn! Oh, well, we'll have to make the sacrifice. It'll be fun going to the Oh Henry again. We haven't been there in a long, long time, and I do love dancing with you, dearest. I'm looking forward to Saturday when I can see you again. I miss you so. I do wish we could be together for always and always. Pretty soon, we will. Right?

All my love and kisses always,

Trude

My one and only forever.

I did drive that night, but shortly after that Trude and I doubled with Russ and his date, Joann, again. He usually had access to his family car without much trouble if we could get gas; with rationing that wasn't always easy. Sometimes we had to scrounge and pool ration coupons for a road trip anywhere. The Paramount Theatre was in Aurora, a nice long ride from Joliet, and a favorite of ours. After the show, we would take the girls to the restaurant at the Baker Hotel, a few short blocks from the movie house, have a snack or something to drink, and then head home.

It was in the back seat of Russ's car that I had one of my more memorable experiences. I placed my arm around Trude's neck and brought her close to me and we were quietly smooching away. At that time of night Russ always had the radio tuned in to the music of the Aragon Ballroom on WGN, so the mood was quite romantic. With the music as background, I felt myself getting more and more excited. While I was kissing her suddenly I felt her tongue slide into my mouth. She French-kissed me! I was taken by complete surprise and pleasure beyond belief. It had never happened before. I almost rose out of my seat as though it had become electrified. I had never had a girl do that to me before.

But she stopped and said quietly in my ear, "How did you like that?"

I could only pant and stammer. I held her closely the rest of the ride home. Where she learned such things, I don't know, but she sure knew how to drive me wild.

May 24, 1943

My darling, Hi, baby mine. I love you, oh, so very much. A million kisses for you from poor me and every one a whopperdoo. How's that? I'm glad you like them.

This will be a terrific weekend. With you 4 days in a row will make life sweeter than sweet and with something to do every evening in a different way will make it wonderful. Agreed? I am anxiously awaiting to see you bedecked in that pretty formal. I like it very much and you look beautiful in it—you do always anyhow, as I have said hundreds of times already.

Could we make a date for Sunday or Monday afternoon or have you other plans? Possibly we could spend both days at the park or swimming. How does that sound? Do hope you will fulfill my desire cause I want to be with you every free moment we have and I hope you feel the same.

I have been looking at a few store windows to see if I could find your surprise—to be presented very soon to you. Thought possibly Chicago's jewelers might provide a better selection but if I don't see anything I like up here, Joliet's resources will have to be honored. I do wish you would let me buy you another ring. Maybe you will change your mind and I am sure you would enjoy the present. I'd buy the best I could, cause the best isn't good enough for my little sweetheart. You will think about it, won't you, honey?

The radio is playing, "Dearly Beloved," and it still is very expressive of my feelings for you, even though the song is a little old. Beautiful—nevertheless—just like you. "It's always you" and you will "Always be in my heart." "Goodnite little Angel" and "I'll see you in my dreams." Bye.

All of my love and,

all of my kisses,

Dick

P.S. Our codes—forever and ever.

xxxxx Wish I could

xxxxx collect right

xxxxx now. Can I

xxxxx collect

xxxxx Wednesday?

The ring to which I referred was an amethyst ring that I got her for her birthday, February 13. I meant it as an engagement ring. She didn't encourage my buying it nor discourage me so I bought it as sort of a temporary ring until with the help of Army pay I was later able to buy a somewhat better diamond replacement.

Trude rarely missed a day writing, but with the demands of medical school being more than I expected, I wasn't always able to write back everyday. I wanted to study when I was alone so that any time I could get away from the books I could spend time with her, rather than write. We were coming up on the anniversary of our first date and we both remembered it fondly.

Tuesday

May 25, 1943

Dearest Darling,

It is 10 o'clock and I am inside as I have been since 8:25 when I returned from the Allerton. I was a good girl & fulfilled your request by not going out walking after 8:30. Heard all of my favorite programs & hear that cute little song, "In My Arms." I'm determined to get a recording of it, and will shop around tomorrow evening (at Wurlitzers, Marshall Fields, & the store on Randolph St.) Do you know of any music stores that might have that particular record? Will appreciate hearing of them.

Sweetheart, I've been thinking of our love affair—good , of course. I think it's really amazing for two to be so very much in love. I'm so terribly happy, my love. I can't seem to wait for our next date, or our next meeting. The time between dates is so very long that it's almost unbearable. I just love to be with you all the time, dearest. And when we're together and the time for parting arrives, I really hate to see you go. If we could only do something about that, (you're not leaving me evenings) I'd be in ecstasy. I guess I'm just afraid to do anything about it—for there is a solution as mentioned in your letter of today.

I'm looking forward to our long and beautiful weekend—4 whole days (sigh). It's going to be wonderful. I do hope the days are warm enough for a picnic. There is nothing I like more than being with you enjoying the sunshine and beauties of nature. In my estimation it would be heavenly.

When I get home Friday nite I am going to check on the dates of our first date (the Senior Ball at Ill.) I'm quite certain it's the same date as the Jr. Col. Formal. We can celebrate and reminisce, for I had a perfect time that eventful and significant day. Wearing the same formal will make it more real. I'm glad, happy, thrilled that it did happen; thankful for the picture in the paper; your first letter and our beautiful love affair. I wonder what would have been the situation if the Herald News photog. hadn't asked me to pose & never would have received your letter.

Goodnite my love. Will dream of you this evening. Remember I'll be loving you every waking moment.

All my love & kisses always,

Trude

May 27, 1943

Darling, dearest Trude,

Tonight is the night isn't it? You and I dancing together the same way we did a year ago. It was a most wonderful evening, wasn't it, honey? The start of a beautiful love affair and I'll bet no one thought it would be that way—except me—I was hoping very much you know that you would be mine always and always.

Now for my poem which came out of my head this afternoon as I sat gazing at your cute picture:

It was only a year ago

That a girl named Trude met her beau.

And what an evening that became

For my heart was never the same.

She is the sweetest girl in all the world

And her love and mine is so encurled

That someday soon she'll be my wife

And to make for her a happy life.

Love affairs are, oh, so swell

And I'm the one who can really tell

Cause to have a girl as nice as Trude

Is something in life that is really cutie.

"I love her," "I love her," I'll shout aloud

And hold my head up in a cloud.

The days ahead will be just grand

Cause she'll be with me—hand in hand.

Now my poem has come to a close
And I know that I can't compare.
But as long as Trude is pleased with it
I'll know that I have made a hit.

I love you my darling and can't wait to see you in your pretty gown. Bye
for now.
All my love & kisses,
"Your one and only forever"
P.S. Our codes always & always.

When we could escape the city we would go home to Joliet and to
a forest preserve nearby. She really liked the walks in the country
although in her letter of June 1, she mentioned the one drawback to
those jaunts:

Our weekend was gorgeous but just too short. Hoped it was just begin-
ning. Yesterday's visit to the woods was luscious except for the bites I
received which are causing a great deal of discomfort today. Dearest, I hoped
yesterday afternoon would never end. It was heavenly lying on the grass
beside you in the gorgeous country. I love you so terribly much that I don't
know what I'd do without you. You seem to give me so very much joy and
happiness. I'm glad I didn't miss all of this. It would have been horrible.

In her letter of June 3, she playfully extolled her skills as a cook, an
important quality in a wife in those days:

Thursday
10:45 p.m.
Dearest, dearest, Darling
I love you, love you, love you, lots & lots & lots. I love you very, very,
very much. I'll love you now and always and always. Love you more than
I've ever loved you in the past. My love for you grows by the day, the hour,
the minute. Pretty soon it will be "Boom" and you know what that will
mean. No- No- No! We'll be married, one-and only love, something we
waited for four years. Right?
Good morning, darling, what would you like for breakfast? Fine, I can
toast bread very well if I have a toastmaster. I'm awfully proud of it. And

coffee, that's simple, even a child can make it. As far as juices are concerned, they can be purchased in cans. That's the best I can do for breakfast.

Now for lunch—would you like baloney or cheese sandwiches. Fine, that's easily done. 2 slices of bread, lettuce or relish or dressing. Also milk, which will do us both good. How was the big lunch? I'm glad you enjoyed it. Incidentally, we could buy a Grennan cake or pie for dessert.

Now for dinner—just a little ride to the Allerton & there we are. No dishes to do, either.

Well, do you still think I'd make such a good wife? Not as far as meals are concerned. You should be convinced by now. You would lose weight instead of putting it on, dearest. Now that you know, you can back out if you wish.

Sorry, dearest, I was just kidding. I'll learn after a while & I'm sure you'll be proud of my cooking. I'll do everything in my power to make you happy & contented.

I missed you so very much today, dearest. By the way, you have a little unknown aid in your plan to change my mind about marriage. It's Dorothy, the newlywed in our department. She knows I am going steady & asked me if we were contemplating marriage in the near future. I told her how I felt & and she thinks I ought to get married as soon as possible, she thinks its loads of fun. Now you have someone plugging with you, on your side. Taint fair—2 against 1.

Goodnite, my love. It's exactly 11 p.m. & bedtime. Will see you at 4 p.m. at Walgreens (inside) on Saturday. It's too long a wait as far as I am concerned. Will be waiting anxiously, sweetheart.

All my love & kisses always,

Trude

P.S. XXXXXXXXXXX (1 for each month)

The "boom" was her fear that one of these nights our impassioned necking would go too far and she would wind up pregnant—a fate worse than death in those puritan times. There were stories about girls who had killed themselves rather than face their father's wrath for the sin of an illegitimate child. I couldn't even imagine that scandal of two pillars of their respective communities—Matt Pisut and Joseph Zalar—having their kids do such a thing. She warned me often of, as she quaintly put it, "Cutting the wedding cake before the marriage."

A "Grennan" cake was one of the products made by the Purity Baking Company that Trude and I both loved. Walgreen's was a large drug store where Trude and I would meet for a Coke or whatever. It was a cheap date, but neither of us had much money. There was always something to do in Chicago, a show or play, a museum or window shopping. A favorite spot most of the year was Oak Street beach, a few blocks from the Girls Club, her rooming house on Michigan Avenue. During the warm months, we would go to Lake Michigan and watch the waves crash against the sea wall, and then slide out with a rush. We talked about everything and nothing until it was time to go.

The War Department did not allow us a summer break, so I continued my schooling, and saw Trude in the city as often as we could manage. We wrote every chance we got, sometimes even right after we had come home from seeing each other.

If we took the streetcar downtown I would ride with her back to her stop, see her home and then get a trolley to my place. Many nights I would linger outside the Franciscan Girl's Club saying goodnight, kissing her, stroking her hair, wishing I didn't have to leave. Some nights we would catch her landlord, the owner of the club, spying on us out the window. I was never sure if it was jealousy, disapproval, or protective instinct that made him keep an eye on us.

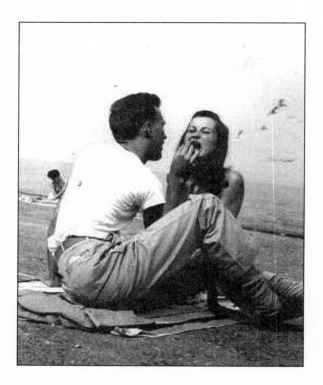

Me applying Trude's lipstick
at the beach. (top)

Stacks and stacks of our
letters.

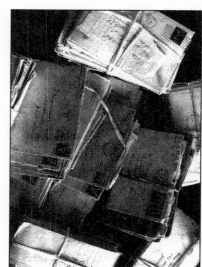

Summer Love Letters

We continued our correspondence that summer with a few little ups and downs but no major events, just our droning on about our humdrum lives and our infatuation with each other.

ETA of Nu Sigma Nu

626 S. Ashland Blvd.

Chicago, Illinois

June 3, 1943

Hi, sweetheart of mine:

Had a nice time last evening, didn't you? We'll have to visit the beach more often and get a good tan. As long as it's becoming warmer every day, we could go swimming on Wednesday's instead of going to the show or to Walgreens, o.k.?

Happy anniversary, honey. A little ahead of time but I can't wait till the day arrives. I've got a poem for the occasion. Want to hear it now? Good.

On June 14th of '42
"Trude," I said "I want you."
Trude replied, "My love is yours"
And I knew then that mine was hers.

She wore my pin and said aloud
"I love you," and my heart did pound.
I kissed her once, I kissed her twice
And every one was oh, so nice.

And now the date is '43
She is mine forever to be.
Love is swell and I'm the man
To make her happy the best way I can.

I love you my sweet and can't wait until the day when I can place a ring
on the third finger of your left hand. Hope it will be soon.

All of my love & kisses,
Dick

June 6, 1943
My Darling:

I just got home and I couldn't wait to write to you after our wonderful,
wonderful evening together. I'm so happy that we're so much in love and
that our wedding date isn't too far off. I hope very much that you will
shorten the 2 years to the very near future so we can be with each other night
and day for always and always.

To have you for my wife will be an honor cause you are so sweet, nice,
and loving. Do wish from the bottom of my heart that you would marry me
right now. You'll consider it deeply, won't you darling? How about surpris-
ing me on our anniversary date with an answer and I'll be the happiest fel-
low in the world.

Hope my proposal was demonstrative of my love for you. Please marry
me soon, honeybunch.

All of my love & kisses,
"your loving husband"

June 7, Monday
4:15 p.m.
Dearest Darling,

I just finished reading your very nice letter. It was so very sweet of you
to write so late in the evening. You're such a dear that I don't know how I'll
stand being unmarried for 2 years. What can we do? I love you so very much
that I feel very sad & blue without you. Really, dearest. I feel lost, as if I'm

lacking something very, very important. I don't have any ambition, I feel very lifeless.

I received a letter from Elaine Webber yesterday. You remember her— she's the girl I worked with at duPonts. She's planning her wedding for June 20 and she'd like me to be a bridesmaid if her husband-to-be can get his 3rd friend out of the army that week. Here's hoping. If he doesn't succeed, she would like me (us) to attend the wedding. I'd rather be a bride, of course, but by being a bridesmaid I'll get into the game, no doubt. Maybe then I'll change my mind a little sooner about things. What is your opinion?

I think your proposal was super. I can't say anything but "Yes" to that, and very soon, also. I don't see how it is possible, dearest. I do wish you would make me see it your way. I can't help but think it very unwise & foolish and I know everyone else sees it my way. We'll talk more about it Wednesday. O.K.? I'd love to.

Goodbye for now, dearest. I love you very very much and want you for my husband, and want you as soon as possible.

With my love & kisses always,

Trude

Obviously getting guys home for leave just when you wanted them was not always easy with war on, so it was in doubt whether her friend's friend would be able to make the wedding.

Monday evening

June 7, 1943

My sweetheart,

I am awaiting your call tonight with anxiety. Every time I hear your sweet voice over the phone, I am in another world. It's so wonderful to be able to talk with you every night and to hear you say, "I love you lots."

What should we do next Monday evening? Anything you desire is all right by me. Think of something extraordinary since it is a special special occasion. I can't wait to give you something you want very much. I do hope you like it very much. Tried to get the best I could with my available resources. When I start making money, with the Army as my donator, I'll be *able to buy things for you more often, since I like to buy you different things to express my heartfelt love.*

Hope you will write to me quite often—I love and enjoy your letters very much. Bye for now. All of my love & kisses,

Dick

P.S. Our codes—forever & ever & ever.

xxxxx I.O.U.

xxxxx Wednesday

xxxxx night

xxxxx signed

xxxxx Dr. R.W. Zalar

Tuesday

June 8th

Dearest Darling Sweetheart,

I feel simply wonderful this evening. You see I'm very very much in love with you and only you—"My Dream of Tomorrow." I do wish you could be with me every evening. I'd love to help you do your studying. It would prove very interesting for me, helping you learn; I'm so bored with myself and my roommate. Aren't I terrible?

Am thinking about calling Viv from work tomorrow & surprising her. This will make up for the letter I'm not going to write to her this week. I haven't seen her since last weekend you know. My days were filled with dates with someone very very dear to me. He's so wonderful that I love being with him every possible moment. He wants me to marry him very soon, and I can't wait for the earliest possible moment to become his wife.

All my love & kisses,

Trude

P.S. Our codes forever & ever, dearest.

Thursday

June 10

Dearest Dick,

Think I'll get to bed early tonite, in about an hour (9:30 p.m. now). I'll have to store up some sleep for our weekend. Right? We'll have 3 big consecutive days and that's really an overdose. I think I would like going to the Edgewater Monday nite. The beachwalk opens soon I am informed and perhaps we can go formal sometime. Russ Morgan is at the E.B. and he's pretty good, isn't he? Am looking forward to Monday nite, dearest. Just know we'll have a wonderful time.

I hope my phone call this evening did not disappoint you too much, that is, our conversation of a matter of great importance. I'm sorry I feel as I do, but today's incident changed my mind definitely against our plans. It is possible that I'll change my mind after a while, but if you don't care to wait, I'll release you from our bargain. I love you very very much, dearest, and I think I always will, but if you don't think I'm being fair by being so changeable you may do as you wish. Don't misunderstand, I don't want to give you up for I love you very much. I always will. But if we can't agree on matters, one should give in or we should give it up. I believe we did discuss this thoroughly this eve. & you decided to wait along with me. We can forget about that for the present.

Sweetheart, I love you & miss you tremendously. I often hope that your educa. be at an end and that you have your degree & title of doctor. I pray for you each time I'm in church & ask the Lord to help you become one of the very best doctors so that I could be proud of you. I never lack confidence and know my prayers will be answered. Don't get discouraged, dear—you'll make it & you know it. I do. I'm sure your mom is helping also so please don't give up. Also you'll be one of the oldest and healthiest M.D.'s alive, so don't think about that, either. I'm not.

Pretty soon we will be very very happy. Let's not rush into things. It isn't very wise.

All my love & kisses,
Trude

July 8, 1943
Dearest darling, sweetheart, lovely one,
Thinking of our being married very soon makes me tingle all over and to know that you will be with me always is a wonderful feeling.

I am going downtown Saturday to get a picture frame for your pictures. They are so pretty and I want to keep them clean and beautiful so that they will be nice for always. Whenever I'm lonely I look at your smiling face and pretend I'm with you and holding you in my arms. Then I feel good—not really, but it helps me anyhow.

I'm breathless, speechless, and just plain "I don't know." It's really wonderful to hear you talk about such nice things as our marriage, love affair, etc.

I send millions of kisses to you and wish September was tomorrow. I'll dream of you tonight and will see you Saturday. Nighty-night sweetie.

All my love & kisses,

Hubby

P.S. Our codes—forever.

P.S. xxxxxxxxxxxxxxxxxxxxxxxxxxxxxxxxxxxxxxxxxxxxxxxxxxxxxxxxxx

Monday

July 12, 1943

Dearest Darling,

I certainly feel very much better since talking to you. Hope it will hold me over until tomorrow night. When you're away I'm just not myself, I'm an altogether different person. I cannot understand myself.

About our marriage, dearest, you needn't ever think that I'll change my mind. I'm as anxious as you, dearest, and can hardly wait. The sooner the better. I don't think we're too hasty, do you?

Either way, we'll have to make a sacrifice—the trimmings if we make the great day soon, 2 years of happiness if we wait. Which would you rather do? The former, of course, as I would.

Of course, it's a responsibility to make things work. Where will we live? Near your work or mine?

Will have to bid you goodnite, dearest. Here's a kiss for you—XX.

All my love & kisses, always,

Trude

July 12, 1943

My Honeybunch:

I've been dreaming again all day long, the thoughts of our wedding in September have been running thru my mind and the more I think of it, the *more certain I am that it won't be wrong to make the step so early in our young lives.*

Anyhow, whatever you want to do is what I want to do and your desires are my commands. I'd buy the world with a fence around it if I was able but I'll have to wait until my first million rolls in, then you will have everything you want, including me, O.K.?

I've got your snapshots on this wall above the desk and they are very nice. I sneak a kiss when you aren't looking. Don't mind, do you? Good.

You are mine and I just want to think of you as my wife from September until ???—end of time—O.K.? Goodnite love of my life. I miss you lots.

All of my love & kisses,
Hubby

August 23, 1943
Monday
My one and only sweetheart:
I am a little lost as to how I should start this love note. It's been so long since I have written, that I hope I haven't lost my poetic ability, but I know I can always tell you of my love and affection.

Your phone calls help so very much my honey and I'm glad that you are so close to me. I think I would have gone crazy, if you hadn't come up here to work. You know how hard it was for both of us not to see each other— only on Saturday when you were home.

Hope that you will be my little wife in a short while.
I feel a poem coming on—can you take another one? Hope so.
"My heart beats faster when I see
That Trude my love wants to be,
My one and only forever & ever.
Her lips I love to kiss, so much
She has the nicest, gentlest touch.
And I love her so very much—
Forever and ever
When she'll say "I do"—"I do"

I know that I'll be in heaven too,
For she'll be mine till we say adieu—
Forever and ever.
Maybe the little ode wasn't too good this time but I hope you like it cause
it's from the bottom of my heart. I love you, Trude, always and always. Bye.
All my love & kisses,
Dick

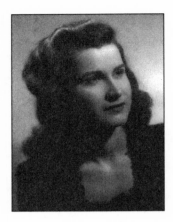

Trude's engagement
photo. (top)

Our wedding photo.

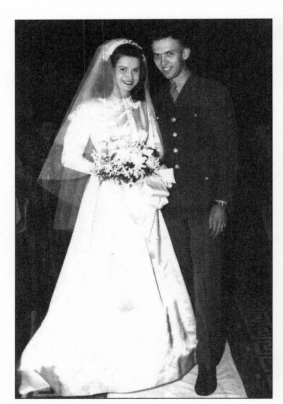

We Set the Date

W hen things were slow at work, Trude found time to type me a note now and then. Things were a lot less hectic at the baking company office and now that she was living in the city, the commute was a lot less time-consuming so she had more time for shopping, and for me.

Part of the reason for waiting to get married was that if we did, we could afford a much nicer wedding than would be possible on what I was making while I was in school at the rank of private first class. After med school, I would be a lieutenant with a significant pay raise. Trude's family couldn't afford to put on a big wedding with all of her younger siblings to feed and clothe, and my family certainly didn't have lots of extra money to spare on a lavish affair.

One of the factors in helping to sway her was when I spelled out our finances. She was always very smart when it came to money, and I decided to appeal to the natural accountant in her in a letter:

I have been figuring as I told you, of how we could spend our money. I'll write it down and you can make your judgment on it—you're the boss. I make $54 a month (pay) and $82.50 (for room and board). Total will be $136.50. But $12.50 goes for a war bond and $6.50 for the $10,000 insurance policy leaving $117.50. Now you make $27.50 a week or $119 a month. Total for both of us is $236.50 a month. (not bad, huh?) If we can get an apartment for $60 a month, food around $50 a month, laundry at $15 a month and accessories such as clothes for you and other things, $70, then we'll have spent $195 which will leave us $41.50 a month for other fun.

*Whoops, almost forgot income tax. We'll have to save for that too. So you
can see we can live very nicely on our paychecks.*

She couldn't find a flaw in my logic and agreed that a wedding
sooner, rather than later, was in order. We set the date for September
16, 1944.

Early in 1944, I moved to an apartment only a few blocks from the
university campus, so going to and from classes was no strain. When
a student entered his last year, the fraternity asked him to find other
quarters to make room for the younger students joining the house.
Clyde Kirchhoff, a fraternity brother and a good friend, moved in with
me and shared expenses.

One advantage of not living in the fraternity house was Trude
could visit me rather than me always going to her place, where we
had no privacy, or someplace out in public where we were also not
really free to neck. Until I moved, I had found myself missing the back
seat of Russ's car. The evening of her birthday in February, she came
back to my place to open her present.

I had purchased pajamas for her from one of the better department
stores in Chicago. I wasn't making much money from the Army, but
liked to spend the little extra I had on her, and she always seemed to
like nicer things for her wardrobe. As she admired the nightwear, I
said, "Why don't you try them on so I can see if they fit and if they do
you justice?"

She was rather nervous about it, but I coaxed her into it. After all, I
had seen her in her bathing suit many times, and the pajamas were
not some flimsy negligee that would reveal more than she did at the
beach. Finally, she relented. I'd never seen her in such informal attire
but when she came out of the bathroom, my jaw dropped. Even
though I was not seeing more of her than I had before, there was
something so risqué about seeing her dressed for bed that it drove me
crazy. She wanted to change back into her clothes immediately, but I
talked her into having a seat. The only place to sit in my small apartment was on the Murphy bed that was always in the down position.
Murphy beds were quite popular in those days and the source of

much humor in slapstick movies of the time. They were beds that were hinged to fold down out of a door, like a closet. This allowed you to have a bed by night and a lot more living space in the room by day. But since it was the only place to sit in my room, my bed was down most of the time.

She sat down and I sat next to her. Soon we were hugging and kissing as though the ship were sinking and this was our last goodbye. As our necking became hotter and heavier, we changed to a prone position on the bed and became more heated with passion.

Suddenly she sat up and pushed me off of her. "We'd better stop. I have to go. It's getting late."

Even though it was late, I didn't want her to leave. But we both feared what would happen if she stayed much longer. She tried to bring me back to reality. "Dick, this is Friday, and we have all of tomorrow and Sunday to be with each other."

I reluctantly agreed as she held my hand. I knew I was soon going to have Trude completely and forever, but seven months seemed an eternity to wait for an excited young man.

Trude changed back into her clothes, and we took the streetcar back to Michigan Avenue and the Girls Club. It seemed like a long ride that night, sitting so close and not being able to touch her anymore. At work the next week, she typed:

Dearest love,

I missed you terribly last night after you left. Slept on my pillow and dreamed of you, love.

Do wish you were here right now—wish I could see you every morning, noon and night from now until always. I would be in 7th Heaven.

Dorothy commented on your picture last night. She thinks you resemble Jimmy Stewart. She thinks that you look so different on your new picture that there is no resemblance to the old one.

I like them both, but I can't quite decide on which you look younger. No matter, though, you look quite sharp in both of them. I am very proud of them both. Lots and lots and lots and lots of love.

Trude

About the time of her birthday, we had gone out to dinner at one of our favorite restaurants on the north side of Chicago. I had wanted to make things official, so after we ate and were enjoying ourselves, I took a small box from my coat pocket and gave it to her saying, "Trude, will you marry me? I bought an engagement ring. I hope you like it."

She looked at me, squeezing my hand that she had been holding and said, as her eyes filled with tears, "Well, I can't say anything but yes. You surprised me a little since I thought we would wait for a while. I'm so happy."

She cried as she unwrapped the small package and opened it. The tears flowed harder as she leaned over the table and kissed me. She asked me to slip the ring on her finger, which I was only too happy to do. It took on a new sparkle on her hand.

On February 17, she found time at work to type another letter:

Thursday

8:25

Dearest Love,

Since it is so very early in the morning, and because yesterday was a very slow day, we are still without work. I am very glad for it gives me an opportunity to surprise you with this letter.

Love Dove, I do want you near me every day of the year and everyday of my life. I know you feel the same, and I just can't wait to make preparations for that great day to come. I will commence immediately in March sometime when you can tell your dad. We can then name the day and that will make things seem more real than ever. Love, do you think you will be very nervous? I hope not, for one of us will have to remain calm and, of course, that one will have to be you.

Believe I will go down shopping this evening. I have in mind to purchase some rubbers, material (I hope), the next issue of the "Bride's Magazine", may look at suits at Rothschild's, and if I have some time, will shop around for a new spring dress. Do you think I will ever be able to save any money?

Since it is so miserable outdoors, I don't believe I would like to go up to Lake Forest this weekend. Now if I had a new formal or dress to wear, it would help matters much. Of course, if you would like to go, I would be

WE SET THE DATE

happy to go also; after all, I do want to please you. Do you suppose Russ and Judy will be terribly disappointed?

I wonder what your dad thought when he saw the picture in the paper. I can hardly wait to hear. Do you suppose he was as thrilled as we were? It makes things seem more true since all the people know of our first step.

Lots of love always,

All my love always,

Trude

Just prior to our engagement announcement appearing in the paper I had told my father of our plans. He knew I was quite serious about her, so the news didn't come as any surprise. My father knew her father's prominent position in their community, which didn't hurt.

A letter in April was typed and came decorated with hearts and cherubs she had cut and pasted on it. I marveled at her creativity and that she would take the time to think of all this.

Thursday

My dearest ittle bittle Dick,

I know it's a little late but I wish to fank ou for the tweetly scented bid box of dutin powder. I used it lat nit and it thur thmelt purty. I no ou tould-n't tmell of the fowder. Tum day I will put on lots of dust for ou, and den ou kin thmell hos purty I tmell.

Tweetheart, I taught the tards were purty too. It was tweet of ou to member me at Easter n I am torry I didn't member you—but I did. The fic-ture of the picnic on 1 tard sure was purty wasn't it, it brot back memries uf hour ittle picnics (no food dough) in de woods, member ast summer. De odder tard was tweet too, but de man's ficture didn't ook ike ou, tause ou are ots more andsome.

De tandy was dood too. I guess ou want me to grow big and fat, don't ou? Well, I tan't cause I'se wean ike ou. and big too. I iked de box de tandy was in. It were very apropos. Tink i ill teep de box and fave it. Now i ave 2 boxes' ready, 1 fum ast ear and 1 from ust ear. Tank ou for de boxes.

Ust 1 more ting. i ike easter bunnies. Do ou tink i tould ave 1 next ear? i ove em so much, most as much as ou. It needn't be a tall bunny ust a ittle 1 ike ou, mith soft fluffy fur.

My boss pays me to werk, so now i must go back to werk. I uv ou very much, and miss ou lots. Soon we will be merred, and den we kin be together.

All my love,

Trude

P.S. i ope ou ad an easier time weading mi note wen I ad witing it for it weally tuk a long time, but I ove ou and ike to spend a long time on ou.

Luv and tisses always fum yer 1 & ownly dirlfriend and wife Trude to my won & ownly boyfriend, fiancée, and husband.

Such craziness of course brightened my tedious days of studying. I wrote back and saw her as often as I could. And counted the days until our wedding.

That summer I had to continue my crammed schooling with no break. Trude and I saw each other as often as possible although she was busy getting ready for the big event. She spent a lot of time to make sure it would be just right. With her living and working in Chicago and having to take the train to Joliet, it was difficult for her to oversee all of the details, but somehow she managed beautifully.

I would join her and try to be of some help when my school and Army obligations permitted. Every Saturday, the classes had to assemble outside the medical school and we would march in formation and learn other routines. Our induction training we had finished months before, but it all was just being re-emphasized, since upon graduation we all were to be officers and leaders. We knew we weren't really going to be combat soldiers, but we were expected to know when to salute, remove our hats, and the other most basic details of military life.

She arranged for the bridesmaids' gowns at a store in Chicago and bought her own gown, which, as tradition dictated, I wasn't permitted to see. She had saved a note from the shop manager that said:

Dear Miss Pisut:

Your dress is of traditional white satin. It has a peter pan collar and capped sleeves, edged in fagoting. The bodice and hooped skirt are gracefully

gathered into a waist-band. This is one of our loveliest colonial style
dresses. We feel sure that you will always treasure it.

Signed, Joan Adair

Our letters became fewer that summer as we spent more time together, and the time we spent apart was too full of activities to leave much time for writing.

A few days before the wedding, I received the last in this string of 347 letters which had allowed us to get to know each other so well and made our love affair possible.

Dearest darling,

I missed you very much this evening. For a minute, I was lost and felt very alone so in order to make time pass I began to do some of my little jobs. I called all the people I could about the breakfast and I have the number down to 50, with four people calling me tomorrow and about four more couples to ask. We'll probably have about 40 people. Next, I sorted my clothes; some for the cleaners, some for pressing. I also made a list of "things to do." I washed my hair and started working on my skirt alterations. I also wrote five thank you notes. I think I'll call it quits for the night.

Incidentally, Viv said that all the people at her house liked the gowns— something different and very beautiful. I feel better now. She thinks my suit, hat, and shoes are adorable too. I feel so much better.

Dearest, I wish you wouldn't study too hard and get all worn out. Remember our big day Sat. I can't wait. I know we will be immensely happy—just you and I in our first little home. It will be like heaven, darling. I love you ever so much and want to be with you every minute, "more than you'll ever know." I love you, dearest. Goodnite, my baby,. xxx. Here's a big kiss for you, my sweet. X

With all my love, Trude

P.S. I love you and miss you very much tonite.

The wedding was held on the morning of September 16, 1944, at Sts. Cyril and Methodius Church in Joliet. It was just a few doors away from where Trude and her family had lived for the past 31 years. Unfortunately, due to the war, many people we would have liked to have join us for the occasion were unable to do so. Her brother Matt was absent, away on duty in some far corner of Asia, as were so many of our friends in the service, and many others who found it impossible to travel with the gas rationing and other restrictions.

The altar and the rest of the church were beautifully decorated. No doubt Trude and her sisters had a lot to do with that. Since her father was a very prominent church member and the funeral director for most of the parishioners, there was a little more effort put forth on everyone's part, and I'm sure he had good relationships with the florist and the other people who were necessary to help make the limited budget look like a million bucks. After all, Trude's first job had been cleaning sacristy floors of the same church when she was in grade school there, so it was understandable that everyone would want to make it look special.

When I arrived a short time before Trude, people were gathered at the bottom of the stairs in front of the church, wanting to get a look at the beautiful bride-to-be when she made her appearance. A large crowd of over 100 relatives, friends, and neighbors was already seated in the main section of the church, with others standing in the rear. She was accompanied by her maid of honor, her oldest sister, Agatha, whom she had kept awake so many nights writing to me, and bridesmaids: one of her younger sisters, Anna Mae, and Vivian Pironciak, her closest friend.

Being in uniform at all times was required during the war so I wore mine with the single insignia on each sleeve identifying my rank. I waited in a side room next to the altar with my oldest brother, Joe, who was the best man, and the ushers—my best friend, Russ Stevens, and Bob Gaspich, a longtime neighbor and friend who had played a crucial role in getting Trude and me together to begin the whole story.

We came out to the altar, and when Trude came into the church on her father's left arm and started to walk down the aisle towards me, it was like the world stopped turning. All eyes went toward her lovely presence. I could barely breathe. I had waited so long for this moment, I wasn't sure I hadn't passed out and was dreaming the whole thing. The organ music filled the church, heightening the drama. As she neared the altar, I came to her, she smiled, extended her right arm, and we walked up the two steps to our positions. We were married at 9:15 a.m.

Snuffy Sanello, the handyman at my sister Marion's home in Joliet, drove us to the La Salle Street station to catch a train to New York for our honeymoon. Although the wedding had been early that morning, by the time the wedding mass, breakfast, the party at a hotel and all of the visiting and last minute details were over, we almost missed the train. We got to the platform at 4:29 and went running for the 4:30 train in a scene right out of a bad Hollywood movie.

It was a16-hour ride to New York. We couldn't afford a sleeping berth which meant we sat up the whole time and tried to nap as well as we could in each other's arms. Propriety being what it was in those days, there wasn't much more than a little handholding along the way. We had five days in New York, staying at the Park Vanderbilt Hotel. As brief as the visit was, we managed to do a lot of sightseeing and went out every night to the Copacabana, Versailles, Latin Quarter and some of the other legendary hot spots of New York. We even made it to the Stardust Room of the Waldorf-Astoria, but due to my lack of savvy in knowing to tip the maitre' d enough, we ended up with a table so far from the action that by the time we started for the dance floor to move to one of our favorite songs, the song was over.

When we went to the top of the Empire State Building, she refused to even look over the edge, way down to the bustling streets far below, she was so intimidated by the height.

Our whirlwind pace of wanting to see all there was of New York had one funny consequence for Trude. It was our first visit to the Big Apple, and we wanted to taste it all. Among the must-see attractions was the Roxy Theater for the movie and the stage show which featured the fabulous drummer Gene Krupa as the headliner. The lights dimmed, and a man was silhouetted against the curtain in an elevated position above the stage floor. And then the sound began—at first it was a slow drumbeat and then the noise grew: he was beating the drums in a swelling crescendo. As the thumping got louder and faster, the rest of the band joined in, and the sound got heavier and louder, the music expanding to fill the large hall. The curtains ripped open revealing Krupa seated at his drums, his sticks blurring through the air as he pounded out the rhythm. The grand entrance had its intended effect, and the audience exploded with clapping, whistling, and shouting. I nudged Trude to see what she thought of this musical extravaganza unfolding in front of us.

She was sound asleep.

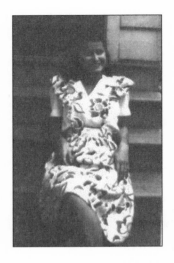

Trude when she was
pregnant with Rick. (top)

Trude, the proud mother with
our firstborn, Rick.

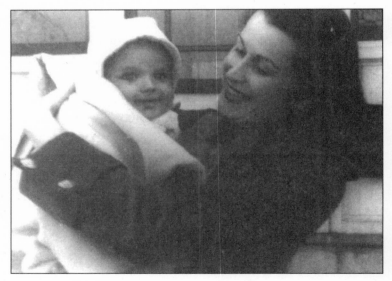

We Become a Family

After our wild time in the city that never sleeps, we slept all the way back on the train and returned to the little apartment I had rented on West Elm Street in Chicago to begin our married life. We were now even closer to our favorite beach and would often take the walk there when time and weather permitted.

We made that little place into our love nest and had to get used to life with each other. I'm sure we had our squabbles, but nothing major even sticks in my memory. Somehow I managed to resist the constant temptation of Trude's presence to study for medical school. The school and the army were really trying to pack a lot into a short time, and Trude made sure I cracked the books when I had to.

The first real fight of our marriage took place because of a visit to my sister Dolores in Cleveland, Ohio, a few months after the wedding. We went to a dinner party with Dolores, her husband and some of his friends. They were all 10 years older than us young newlyweds. An orchestra was playing, and Trude was asked by one of my brother-in-law's friends, "Snitz," to dance. She said, "Yes." As I watched them move about the floor to the strains of this and that tune, Trude seemed to be extraordinarily close to this "older man." I even thought she may have been encouraging him a little too much. I seemed to be a young, immature lad, a little out of place with such a beautiful woman in a sheer, tight-fitting black dress and high-heeled shoes dancing with this suave mature guy. When the laughter and the smiling between them was over and the "thanks" to me was said, she sat back down next to me at the table. I looked at her with dismay, and she knew what I was feeling. I was wondering if I had made a mistake marrying Trude. Who was I to think I could match her flirtatious ways and desires?

On the way back to Chicago, I told her I wasn't happy about the way she had acted, and she said, "I was just teasing him."

I replied, "Well, you're married to me now, and you shouldn't be playing with guys like that." I remembered how she used to tease me about other guys in our letters and wanted that sort of thing to stop completely now that we were married. I'm not sure how much was flirting and how much was just Trude being Trude—all smiles and charm, without a thought as the effect this might have on the guy with whom she was dancing—or what it might do to me.

She did not take my complaint very seriously—clearly the dance meant nothing to her and she couldn't understand my getting so jealous—and this made me angrier. I said almost nothing on the rest of the long trip across the state of Indiana.

She never danced or flirted with anyone again, but I guess I always did feel a bit insecure beside such a beautiful woman and still tended to get a little jealous if anyone paid too much attention to her, although I'm sure there was never any real reason for concern along these lines. Maybe it was good we had that fight rather early so we set some of the ground rules for curbing her behavior and my petty jealousy before it went on long enough to do any real damage.

In June, 1945, I graduated from medical school and started my internship at Garfield Park Community Hospital on the west side of Chicago. I knew when I completed it that I'd be assigned wherever the army chose to send me, which could be any of its many far-flung bases throughout the world. But first I had to attend Fort Sam Houston service school in Austin, Texas, an eight-week course from October to December, 1946, for medical department officers.

Given the places I might have been sent, Madigan General Hospital, in Tacoma, Washington, servicing Fort Lewis and the Second Infantry division, wasn't such a bad place to go. Trude knew this was coming and cheerfully helped pack our meager belongings to have the army truck them across country for the start of our new life. She had done so little traveling in her life that the chance to go anywhere was met with a sense of adventure.

My first assignment as Lieutenant Zalar was in a psychiatric unit for soldiers suffering from anything from simple to quite severe mental problems. This was certainly not the area in which I had wanted to specialize, but this was to be my only really first-hand experience with dementia, and I would find myself grateful for it years later.

Trude got in a family way rather quickly while I was doing my internship, but the first two pregnancies didn't last beyond six weeks. As upsetting as I am sure these miscarriages were to her, she said little to me about them, and I could only guess how she was feeling. A woman simply did not discuss womanly things with her husband, even if her husband was a doctor. The timing would have been bad for a child while I was still in school or interning, so the loss was not as devastating as it might have been.

Once we were settled in Washington, we both felt ready to start a family, and when she again became pregnant she wanted to do whatever it would take to keep this baby. She was worried that whatever had gone wrong before would continue to plague her. Her doctor was being very strict in what she could do and what she couldn't do. He required her to make regular office visits to get shots of hormones that were to protect her from losing this baby.

She followed his orders to the letter, and I was glad she responded to the treatment and that she stayed well as the baby continued to develop on schedule. During the last month of her pregnancy, her weight started to climb, which wasn't totally unexpected, but when she reached the 20-pound limit her doctor had imposed, he wanted to change her diet to make sure she didn't overdo it. One of the goodies he wanted to ration was her daily draw from the plum tree in our back yard. She had been eating eight plums a day and seemed to always be at the tree, as the supply seemed limitless. I had a hard time resisting more than a few a day myself and was having an even harder time trying to keep her from having more than her quota.

I often had to say to her, "You have to watch those plums, dear, or you're going to go over the limit very soon. Only two plums a day and no in-between meals munching." Somehow she managed to stay at the recommended weight.

On the night of September 9, 1947, we were at the theater on the Naval base enjoying a movie when she noticed a twinge of pain in her belly. She didn't react too much, but she whispered to me, "I think it's time. I think I just had a labor pain."

I asked, "Are you sure, dear? Maybe the pain will quiet down or go away. Maybe we should wait a while. I don't want to go to the hospital too soon and then find out this may not be the real thing."

"They're real, and I feel a pressure down below. Let's go now and be sure."

I had yet to learn what all doctors know: that a woman's intuition is rarely wrong. I took her word for it, and we left the theater quickly and headed to the Marine Hospital, a mile away. Trude was always a strong-willed person, and her tolerance for pain was high, and if she said something was happening, I believed her.

I was as nervous as could be, worrying and wondering what the next few hours would bring, not as a doctor, but as any expectant father would be. Even though I had delivered numerous babies during my training program, this was my Trude who was now on the table and all of my training seemed moot. As the hours passed into the morning, the labor pains stayed steady, and I kept questioning the attending physician, trying to get an idea of what was going on. I suppose I made a pest of myself and proved the old saying that doctors make bad patients. He consoled her and me by telling us this was common for first-pregnancy labor and there was nothing to be concerned about. I just held her hand with each contraction and encouraged her to push as she went through the ordeal and occasionally dabbed her forehead with a cool cloth. The father was usually not welcome in the delivery room, so I guess I was lucky to be allowed to stay as long as I was, but once the main event really got going, doctor or not, I was exiled to pacing the waiting room with the other nail-biting fathers.

She took it in stride, but her pain ordeal was quite long. Her doctor stuck with her, carefully monitoring the 26-hour labor. Finally, at 1:30 a.m. on the 11th, Richard Wayne Zalar, Jr. weighed in at 7 pounds, 12 ounces and 22 inches.

Trude was understandably exhausted and drained from the long trial. When the nurse brought our new baby boy out for us to see, his face appeared a little shriveled, as if he hadn't had enough food while he was growing inside his mother. Trude said he looked awfully thin. I thought about the plum tree and said, "Babe, maybe you should've kept eating those plums."

Ten days later, she and Rick had gained enough strength so that I could take her home. She had recovered to almost normal, except for a sore "bottom," as she referred to her own anatomy. She had to be cut, as first-time mothers usually are, in order to ease the baby's entry into this world.

We were in the Northwest, far from family or any close friends, and caring for our newborn was quite a task at first, with no one to turn to for help. I usually fed the baby at night so she could rest a few hours, and during the day, she coped somehow. I know she often wished her own mother were nearby for moral support or to answer questions. Long-distance phone calls were too expensive for her to be able to make them home often.

I can still hear her singing the lovely song "Lullaby" while Rick was going to sleep in his bassinet. She would sit beside him, caressing his head or his cheek or his small hand, assuring him she was always there.

In late 1947, I was reassigned to Fort Sheridan in Illinois, and although the move with a newborn was tricky, we were glad to be coming back home and be within easier reach of our families. Sheridan was 60 miles north of Joliet, near Chicago. At first we stayed at my father's house, and I made the long commute to work. But one night shortly after our arrival, my father scoffed at Trude's cooking, a slight both she and I took very personally, and I decided to quickly find an apartment closer to the base where we could establish our own household. My sister Vida had run Poppa's house and done the cooking a certain way for a long time, and there wasn't room for two chefs in that kitchen. Vida had worked for my father at the KSKJ for about 10 years, but shortly after my return to Illinois, Vida moved to Cleveland to work for our sister in her gift shop there—a job Vida kept for over 40 years.

When Rick was 15 months old, he received an early Christmas present—a new sister. Trude delivered Barbara Judy after only three hours of labor on December 22, 1948. Judy came into this world at 6 pounds, 11 ounces. and 19 inches. Judy and Ricky were precious additions to our lives, and Trude managed to care for the two little ones with the skill of a seasoned juggler. They grew so fast that it seemed the only way possible to record their baby days was with photos.

After I had completed the time I owed the Army and was discharged, I went into practice in the city of Chicago and its suburbs. We were able to put a down payment on a small bungalow in Forest Park, a suburb of Chicago, and we lived there from 1948 till 1951. It was a nice place because there were so many young couples having children and trying to raise them correctly according to either Grandma's rules or Dr. Spock, the famous pediatrician whose book was the gospel for raising kids.

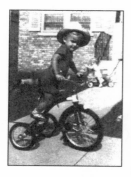

Rick on his trike with Judy playing in the background. (top)

Rick, Judy and Trude at a birthday party.

Me on a ride with the kids at Disneyland.

Trude in all her splendor going out on the town.

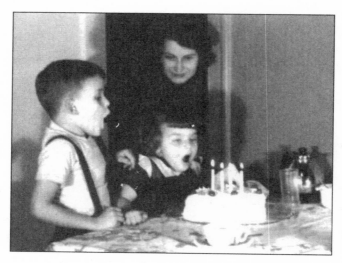

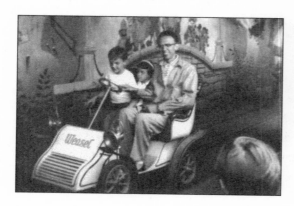

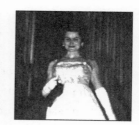

Life in Suburbia

Our life settled into the pattern of so many young couples—so much so that, looking back on it, it almost seems a Norman Rockwell painting viewed with the soft focus of time that takes the sharp edge off the more trying times. Like any new parents, we had our ups and downs, but some things that seemed terrible at the time, became humorous in retrospect.

One warm summer morning when Rick was 3 years old, he gave Trude quite the fright. She let him out to ride his tricycle while she attended to her chores. A short time later she brought Judy out and sat her in her stroller. Trude looked around for Rick, but he was nowhere in sight. She began to call to him but got no answer. She started up the sidewalk, asking the neighbors if they had seen him, and with each negative response, she grew more nervous. No one had seen him. She began to wonder if she should call the police.

The farther from our house she got, the more panicked she became, calling "Rick? Ricky? Where are you?" A block away were the railroad tracks, and she was terrified at the thought of him trying to cross them, maybe a wheel of his trike getting caught in the rails.

As she crossed to the next block, she thought she saw a child on a tricycle ahead of her on the sidewalk. She ran as fast as she could toward him and was disappointed when the startled strange boy looked around. The next stop was the railroad tracks. And just about to cross the rails was a boy on a tricycle. She yelled again, "Rick? Ricky!"

The boy on the bike turned around, surprised to see his mother running at him. When she got to him, she grabbed him and held him tight. Her tears were a flood of joy and relief. She demanded, "Where are you going?"

"I want to see the trains. Can I?"

"All right, but only this one time. No more."

After the visit to the tracks and seeing a train at a safe distance, they headed home. I heard about it in detail at lunchtime. Rick never repeated the trip.

Our daughter, whom the family called by her middle name, Judy, also had an incident on her tricycle when she was 3 years old, and sadly it didn't end as well as Rick's adventure. While riding on our driveway, she fell from her tricycle and severely fractured her skull. She was unconscious and for 24 hours, I sat by her bedside and cried. When she woke up, she was partially paralyzed. A long period of recovery and consultation with every specialist I could find followed. She patiently put up with all the poking and prodding by various doctors and did get better, but always had a few lingering difficulties.

In many respects we were living the typical suburban post-war life. Mom stayed home and Dad worked. Trude had brains, talent and charm, which a generation later would have made her CEO of some corporation, but in those days very few women would have thought of those possibilities.

When I started my practice I made house calls. If someone called about a sick child at 2 a.m., I didn't refer them to an emergency room; I got up and got dressed and went to see the child. I was a perfectionist with my patients, and that sometimes made me a bit of a nuisance at various hospitals, where I was known to be rather demanding. But it made my patients love me, since they knew I was always willing to put out my best effort on their behalf, even if that meant fighting bureaucracy to do it.

I made the money, and Trude made more money with it. I had no luck with the stock market or investments and lost money almost every time I tried. She was good at these things, and I'm sure she more than doubled our money in the market. She had a lot more business sense than I did, so I just trusted her judgment in such things. Years later, when the kids were a bit older, she took a class in investing and did better than anyone in the class with her stock picks.

Trude got pregnant again in 1953, but once again the baby didn't make it to full term. We had moved to River Forest in 1951 and took on a large burden of paying off a 4,200 square-foot eight-room mansion. This village was quite similar to those that dotted the north shore of Chicago: Wilmette, Winnetka, and Lake Forest. Life in the "burbs" was so predictable that William Whyte used nearby Park Forest as the model of conformity in his classic 1956 book, *The Organization Man.*

Life was very orderly—some might now look back and call it regimented. Nowhere was this more apparent than Illinois, which, viewed from the air is a flat, orderly grid of farms. Chicago itself is laid out in a neat north-south, east-west pattern. Our son joked that Greenwich could set its clocks by the precision with which my mother had dinner on the table every night at 6. Trude was very organized and liked things to run smoothly and on time.

Like most post-war baby boom parents, Mom ran the household and, in typical Ozzie and Harriet or Dick Van Dyke fashion, when Dad came home from work, we all took our places at the table, and Trude would ask about my day. Rick once joked about this as "Marcus Welby comes home to dinner." A few nights a week, I would usually have to leave again at 7 to make my rounds at the hospital or go back to the office.

Trude and I had our tiffs, like any couple, but nothing serious, and most of them revolved around my being late to dinner or forgetting to call if I wasn't coming home at all. She went to such trouble to make a nice meal; I couldn't blame her for being upset when I didn't have the courtesy to call. Come to think of it, it was my tardiness that was the source of most of our fights when we were dating, too. When she was really angry about one of these repeated offenses, she wouldn't speak to me for a day or two. If I tried to kiss her good night, she would break her silence only to say, "Get away from me." She could be touchy about certain things and cried easily over small things, going back even to our first exchange of letters, when I had invited her to the fraternity party and then had to rescind the invitation. She knew the tears always worked, and I would melt and apologize profusely for whatever I had done to make her unhappy.

We may have moved to a higher standard of living than we could really afford, and at times we wondered whether we had bitten off a little more than we could chew, but I wanted Trude and the kids to have the best of everything. My Dad's organization, the KSKJ, had a mortgage plan for its members that called for a 10-year note. We paid the money back on time, although it kept things a bit tight, and my income just covered expenses.

With the move from our little bungalow to this home in River Forest, Trude wanted the services of an interior decorator who worked for one of the known furniture stores in Chicago to help set up the new house. I could never refuse anything she really wanted, so she and the decorator planned the details so family and guests always thought the house looked great.

The staircase to the second floor was wide and grand, with a beautifully carved wooden railing. There were 20 carpeted stairs leading to a small landing area where three casement windows faced the northern sky. Bright-colored drapes on those windows caught visitors' eyes as they entered the front hall. At the windows there was a turn and three more steps up to the bedrooms.

River Forest was a gracious community of about 13,000 residents. It had some rather impressive homes, some of which were valued at a hundred thousand dollars or more even in 1951, and certainly would sell for over a million today. One had 26 rooms and looked more like a hotel than a residence—it even had a bowling alley.

Shortly after we moved to this large home, I suggested to Trude that she might want to call an agency to find someone to help with the cleaning as so many people did in those days in that neighborhood. When I got home one evening for dinner, I asked how everything went and how the woman she had hired worked out. Trude told me bluntly the woman would not be returning. When Trude gave her the day's schedule, she told Trude she didn't wash windows. Trude said, "Well, I can sweep and dust!"

The community had schools, churches, and parks with some small stores on the edge of town, but no large businesses to disturb the serenity. It was a nice place to live, and we stayed there for 27 years. We watched our children grow and adjust to a new neighborhood. Rick and Judy received an excellent education at the local public elementary school, half a block from our home on Jackson Avenue. Eventually, Rick went on to high school in nearby Oak Park; Judy stayed closer to home, attending a Catholic girls' school.

Part of our routine was to go down to Joliet almost every Sunday to visit my father and various other relatives and friends. Most of these visits would end up at Trude's parents, where aunts and uncles and lots of other people would stop by. The Pisut house was always a lively place, with various relatives coming and going, and Rick and Judy got to play with their cousins and spend time with their grandparents.

In 1956, we took a car trip West which everyone seemed to do in those days—one major adventure to show the kids America. Rick was 9 and Judy 8 when we set out in a blue and white Oldsmobile convertible with no air conditioning for three weeks. Cruising along Route 66 with the wind in our hair made up for the lack of A/C, and the kids had a ball. In three weeks, we wanted to see and do it all, visiting my college roommate Gordon Sauer, his wife, Mary Lou, and their growing family in Kansas City. On the return trip we spent time in Des Moines with an Army colleague, Bill Morrissey, his wife MaryAnn, and their daughter. Out West we hit the Painted Desert and Grand Canyon. In Southern California we went to a new attraction which had only been open for a year or so—Disneyland. We then visited friends in Carmel, Ventura, Los Altos, and San Francisco, then went to Yosemite, Boise, Yellowstone, the Black Hills, the Badlands and back through Iowa—all in three weeks! The kids loved it and talked about the trip for a long time after we returned.

That same year, Rick and Judy started taking piano lessons with a local teacher, Mr. Amo Capelli, who came to our house. Trude soon became quite intrigued and decided to learn as well. She seemed to have a natural talent for it, and soon she progressed to more advanced songs.

During the holiday season of that year, we invited Jack and Ann Phalen to join us at a special affair at the exclusive Palmer House which was being held by the hospital where I worked. I can still remember Trude coming down the stairs of our house looking like Jackie Kennedy with her gown fitting to perfection, her diamond earrings glistening in the overhead stairway light, her white, elbow-length gloves adding that something extra, and her smile out-flashing the diamonds. A full-length white coat capped off the scene. She absolutely glowed.

The Palmer House was such a Chicago landmark; it's difficult to imagine the city without it. Trude and I had been here before to either enjoy a fine dinner in the renowned Empire Room with dancing to live music between courses or to have a few cocktails with friends in the lounge where Frankie Masters played the piano with his popular orchestra. I remembered it fondly from my dating days as the place to really impress a girl.

Griff Williams, whom we had seen before and very much enjoyed, provided the entertainment for the hospital social, dancing around the stage in front of his orchestra, flailing his baton wildly as he whirled in front of the band, enticing the patrons to join in the fun and get up to dance.

The hotel did everything right, with even the parking attendant dressed in splendid fashion in a long coat with gold buttons and wearing a cap. After he opened the doors, we walked down a long hall leading to the lobby, large chairs lining each side as we approached the staircase. The Beaux Arts ceiling always amazed Trude, and she'd nudge me to look up. It was all quite impressive, especially if your usual date was a drive-in after a movie.

In the ballroom, large crystal chandeliers sparkled above, and the tables were beautifully set with flowers and candles arranged for very striking effect. The night of the hospital formal, after we were all seated, the food was served, starting with the soup. I took a spoonful and made a face. I blurted out to Trude, "This soup is cold." I raised my hand to signal the waiter, but Trude pulled my arm down.

She whispered in my ear, "Dick, this is vichyssoise. It's supposed to be chilled."

Feeling completely foolish, I waved the waiter away. How she learned about things like vichyssoise, I had no idea, but she always seemed to have the right answer. She always wanted to learn how to do things right, so spent a lot of time reading. Of course, I could have read the same thing and still not known vichyssoise when I tasted it.

In '57, we went to Canada, but I was not crazy about flying, so we took the train to Banff, Lake Louise, and Jasper with our good friends Tony and Flo Malone and their children. The next year we took the train to Sun Valley, Idaho, where the adults golfed and the kids played in the pool. The stars in the night sky above Idaho were so amazing that when we got back Trude and Rick took up astronomy as a hobby, checking out books from the library and studying the night sky.

In 1959, we went back to Idaho, this time with Russ Stevens' family as well as the Malones. Russ had not married any of the girls he was dating seriously when Trude and I were dating; he had settled down with another lovely lady, Jean Kelly. It was nice when we'd vacation with another family—Judy was so quiet that she and Rick really didn't have much in common when it came time to play, so having other kids along made it more pleasant for both of them.

Trude's younger sister, Ann, and her husband, Jack, were very much into fishing in Canada. Sometimes we'd go with them, and often in the summer Ann and Jack would go for a week or two by themselves and leave their three kids with us, making for a much more noisy and boisterous household than we were used to. But it was fun and livened things up for Rick and Judy. It also made us appreciate the peace and quiet when they left. It gave us a fun glimpse of what life would have been like had we been able to have a few more children, as we had hoped.

In 1961, we went to Shawnee on the Delaware in eastern Pennsylvania. There was not much to do there except relax, but it had a pool and that was all the kids cared about. One summer we went to Washington, D.C., and had a great time showing the kids—and ourselves—the country. At some point these sorts of long summer trips stopped as the kids got old enough to have other summer activities.

To complete our picture of suburban bliss for those years, of course we had to have a dog, and although we bought our Cocker Spaniel for Rick and Judy, Kippy soon adopted Trude as her pillow. Trude would read the newspaper, and Kippy would rest against her. The dog rarely moved from Trude's side, and after my evening office hours, when Trude would get up to greet me when I got home, Kippy would join her at the door. I'd then plop in the other soft chair and we'd talk about what happened with the kids and anything else, and Kippy would curl up next to Trude again.

Trude took an active interest in our children's activities when they went to Roosevelt elementary. She served as a leader for Judy's Brownie troop and a den mother for Rick's Cub Scout pack. One year she marched with the Cub Scouts in River Forest's annual Memorial Day parade. After the contingent of honored war veterans came the boys in their blue and gold scout uniforms and Trude beside them in her matching uniform. She gave a proud wave to me and the home movie camera as she passed by.

We enjoyed taking movies, and before long we had hundreds of feet of film of all types of get-togethers, family, friends, Rick playing sports, Judy in her Brownie uniform and just about every other conceivable activity. We also took lots of slides and have boxes of them from all of our holidays and travels. Now I'm glad I have all of these to remind me of happier times.

When he was in junior high school, Rick was able to walk home every day for lunch, and this private time he had with Trude forged a special bond that lasted as long as she lived. They could talk about anything.

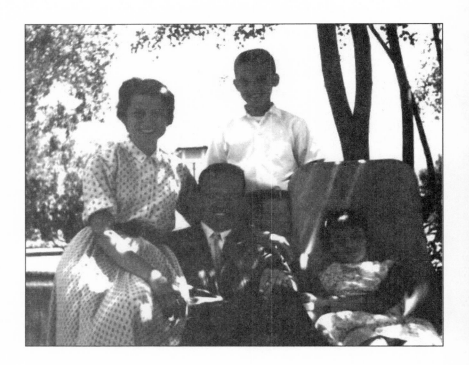

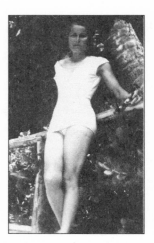

The family at Sun Valley. (top)

Trude at Shawnee on the
Delaware, 1961.

The Sixties

After watching the 1960 Winter Olympics, broadcast on television from Squaw Valley, California, the whole family—in fact, many of our friends and much of the country—got interested in skiing. Later that year we went to Michigan to try the sport for the first time. A couple of years later, over Christmas break 1962, accompanied by the Malones, we took our first serious ski vacation to Sun Valley, Idaho. The comparative cost was very cheap back then because the accommodations were quite simple—just bunk beds in a chalet, and no fancy meals in plush restaurants or staying in chateaus—the point to which things quickly progressed when the popularity of skiing started making it expensive.

I always liked skiing. It's the only sport in which other people sincerely want you to do well and are sympathetic. If you miss a putt in golf, they are secretly glad because now they might beat you, at least on this hole. If you fall down while skiing, they're genuinely concerned and worried that you might have broken something. And they encourage you to do well so you can at least keep up with them.

Sun Valley is a very nice ski area and had some runs that were just right for us rank amateurs, but as our skiing skills improved, we wanted to move on to whiter pastures and started going to Colorado. The slopes in Aspen were a little more difficult, and we needed to learn to ski a little better if we were going to brave these runs, so Trude and I started taking lessons from their experts. She was naturally better than me so was in the more advanced class while I was relegated to the group on the bunny slopes.

One day, as the sun started down, my class headed back to the base of the hill and the ski patrol shack where I was supposed to rendezvous with Trude. I didn't see her anywhere. After waiting and pacing a while, I started to get worried. I went into the ski-patrol office and was told she was in the first aid room. I hurried over there, imagining the worst. Inside, a frightened-looking Trude was lying on a table. She told me the class was learning how to traverse a slope and her leg slipped outward, causing her to fall with her right knee bent away from the slope. It hurt so badly that she couldn't get up, so the ski patrol was called, and they brought her down the mountain on their sled. These sleds always looked fun, but I never wanted to ride one since the only way to earn a ride was to be injured. I checked out her knee. It was apparent she wouldn't be doing any more skiing this trip. I helped her back to our room in the lodge.

The injury ended our winter vacation, and we got the first plane home. When we got back, I contacted an orthopedic surgeon who happened to live nearby. He agreed she had a bad sprain that would take about two months to heal with daily home heat treatments. Each day I would apply heat, gently massage the swollen area, and then rewrap her knee with an elastic bandage. She leaned on my shoulder whenever she had to go anywhere. This same leg would give her trouble in her later years, and I was never sure if it had anything to do with this fall or not.

By the late '70s we were skiing in Colorado regularly enough to buy a condo in Aspen. We kept it until 1985. We were only able to use it a couple of weeks in the winter and for a couple of weeks in the summer, and the rest of time we rented it out. We enjoyed the skiing, and in the summer, the golfing. The mountain scenery was spectacular in either season, and it was fun to rub parkas with locals such as John Denver.

As the kids were getting older and off doing their own things, Trude had more time to explore other things. She won a trophy for bowling on the Riverside Country Club team for the 1959–1960 season. She modeled at fashion shows at the country club and was on the committee for various functions there. In 1965, she won its Class C golf championship. She was also an active member of the auxiliaries at the hospitals where I worked.

It was in the early '60s that she took the investing course and did the best in her class at picking stocks, and later, when it came to playing the market with real money, she always came out ahead

She also became interested in learning how to paint. A friend who lived close to us in River Forest asked her to join the Women's League Club art class. One of the courses was in portrait painting. The teacher was affiliated with Rosary College in town and had quite a good reputation. Trude enjoyed looking at books such as *The Treasures of the Louvre, The Encyclopedia of Art,* and *Three Hundred Years of American Painting* and getting to know the work of major artists. I encouraged her to join the class and try her hand.

She always had a good eye for art, and occasionally we'd go to the fine arts store in downtown Oak Park, a few minutes from our house. Over the years we probably purchased a half-dozen works—both originals and prints. We'd also make trips to the museums in Chicago where we'd admire the work of the great artists.

Trude's drawings still decorate several rooms in our house. None would be mistaken for the work of a master, but they show real skill. One drawing of Rick is a perfect rendition, and the one of me, although unfinished, is also a good likeness. A self-portrait she did is, unfortunately, also incomplete. There are the usual still-lifes of flowers and vases, all of which show a very good raw talent. She just seemed to have a natural sense for proportion, perspective and color.

I still marvel at the painting she did of our home in River Forest. She captured every detail, including the dark red of the brick and the green of the fir tree that guarded the front entrance. I can just see her sitting on a camp chair in the driveway, wearing a bright-colored smock, a beret on her head, an easel in front of her and the tubes of oil paints in the steel case at her feet.

She never really got excited about classical music, but she tolerated my love of opera and always did thoughtful little things to make me happy. Living behind us in River Forest was an older gentleman who owned a music-publishing firm in downtown Chicago. I knew him only in passing—we might talk over the backyard fence as he weeded his vegetable garden and I did yard work. I relished these chats as an opportunity to share his vast musical knowledge. When I was in grade school, my father and I made it a Saturday habit to listen to the Texaco Opera program which, via the still somewhat new magic of radio, brought the greatest voices of the day into our living room. I knew a little about the singers and orchestras who graced the Metropolitan Opera House stage and was always happy to learn more about them from my neighbor.

One Saturday when I returned home, Trude was in the sunroom. After I kissed her and we talked for a few moments about the errands I had done, she took me by the hand, led me to the breakfast room and asked, "What do you think?"

On the table was a pile of 10 records.

"Where did you get these?" I asked in amazement. Eight of them were songs by Enrico Caruso, the famous tenor, singing such famous arias as "Pagliacci," "Vesti la giubba," "Chantique de Noel," "Viene Sul Mar," "Aida-Celeste Aida," and others. The first of these recordings was from 1893. One other was by the German soprano Ernestine Schumann-Heink singing her famous rendition of "Stille Nacht, Heilige Nacht," recorded in 1903. Another was a Sousa Band march from 1903. Curiously, the Caruso albums were recorded on only one side of the very heavy plastic used by the Victor Company back then.

I was speechless for a while as I again sorted through this unbelievable treasure trove. Finally, I asked again, "Dear, where did you get these?"

"At Mr. Forster's house sale. I saw in the paper they were having an estate sale at his house and I decided to go."

Our kindly old neighbor had died a few weeks previous. I had seen him in his garden shortly before his death and thought he didn't look well, but his death still came as an unwelcome surprise.

"Since he died, everything was for sale, and when I saw those old recordings, and knew you were so interested in the old classical opera singers, I couldn't pass up the opportunity. Do you like them?"

"And how! These are priceless, and to hear these voices from way back will be something. I didn't even know such recordings existed." After listening to the recordings, I really wished Fred Forster was still around so I could ask him the story behind these albums, which I felt certain he would have known.

While in high school, Rick studied the derivation of words, and Trude, as she so often did, took an interest in learning new things. She came to enjoy etymology after looking at his textbook and talking to him about the course. She had fun using unusual words such as Sebastian, which meant venerable, and occephalic, which meant egg-headed. She would throw in a fancy word during dinner conversation just to see whether I understood.

Rick was a popular student, good at athletics, and got good grades. As co-captain of the track team, he ran, did the hurdles, and high-jumped. His picture frequently appeared in the local paper for various achievements. He looked at Stanford as well as Yale, but decided on the latter. Of course it made us proud that the Zalars and Pisuts had spanned the distance from blue-collar immigrants to the Ivy League in just two generations.

We took Rick to start school in Connecticut and then went on to Martha's Vineyard for a vacation. Rick did well in college, as well, and upon graduation in 1969 was cited for his efforts in helping the old college make the transition to a co-ed university. They made it sound altruistic, but maybe he just wanted to meet more girls.

After attending Rick's graduation, we went to Hawaii for a couple of weeks. Slowly we seemed to be hitting all of the states. Rick went on to medical school at Northwestern University, in Chicago, and chose as his specialty obstetrics/gynecology.

Judy had some trouble in school and was much quieter generally. I guess Rick took after me and did most of the talking, and Judy took after her mother and was more reserved. Trude's desire to learn new things I think inspired Judy to work hard at her studies in spite of some of the obstacles she faced. I may have been the one with the degrees, but Trude was the smarter of the two of us. Judy started college at a small private school, West Virginia Wesleyan. Her high school counselor in River Forest thought she should try a smaller school with fewer distractions, and Buckhannon, W.V., certainly qualified, but she was not able to complete her studies there. She picked up a few more credits closer to home at Rosary College. Then, years later, with the encouragement of her husband, Ron, Barbara Judy made us proud by completing a degree in psychology at Loretto Heights College in Denver, Colorado.

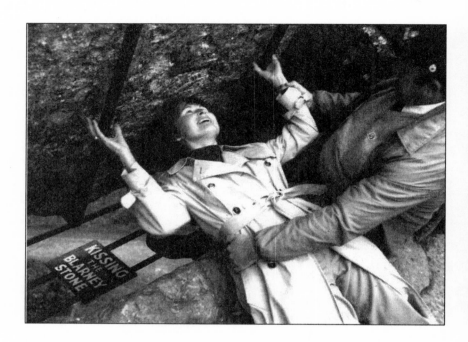

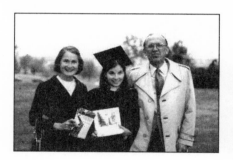
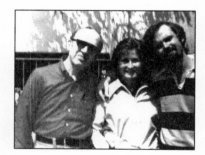

Trude laughing as she kisses the Blarney Stone. (top)

At Judy's college graduation in Colorado. (left)

Me, Trude and Rick, 1975 (right)

That Seventies Time

Trude was an amazing woman whose talents spanned such a broad range of interests and skills. I remember a trip we took to Canada in 1972 with her father and brother—she out-did us all by catching 27 fish the first day. Her father wasn't very happy, since he netted zero for the day. He thought she cleaned out the lake and there wouldn't be any left for him.

This woman who could be so happy roughing it with the boys and fishing was the same one who could set a table worthy of Martha Stewart when we'd have our monthly dinner dates with my doctor friends and their wives—the Malones, Pantones, Irishs and Murphys. She knew all the little touches, like which spoon went where and which fork to use first. She always sparkled as much as the crystal and silver on her table. The women were always impressed by the presentation, the men by the food. She had a vibrant smile and pleasant laugh which came out when one of the guys got to telling stories, but she had a hard time finding a chance to say much when Tony Malone or I or one of the other guys got wound up.

Trude was always a tea drinker and had the dainty qualities usually associated with that pastime. I had read that drinking tea was associated with traditional traits that a woman was supposed to have in those days: "quietness, decorum, and the consumption of watercress sandwiches." I don't think I ever saw Trude actually eat a watercress sandwich, but the rest of the attributes applied. If she was at the country club, the hospital auxiliary, a special charity luncheon, or just lunch with me, she always had to have her tea and held her little finger correctly curled as she lifted her cup. The man who ran our local gourmet tea shop, Bill Todd, used to say, "There are a lot of closet tea-drinkers," but Trude drank hers proudly.

A lot of couples we knew did their own things—he would go fishing or golfing while she went shopping or played bridge. Trude and I liked to do things together, including golfing. When I was around to help clear the table and do the dishes I would, just so we could spend more of our limited time together. Trude always tried to find things for us to do together—if one of us didn't like an activity or couldn't do it, then we found something else to do.

After years of teaching and then director of medical education at St. Joseph's Hospital on the North Side of Chicago, in 1972 I changed jobs and became Vice President of Medical Affairs at a new hospital opened by St. Mary's on the West Side. Supposedly, I would still have time to see patients, but meetings, office politics and other petty bureaucratic trivialities seemed to consume most of my time. After three years, I returned to doing what I became a doctor to do—treating the sick—not shuffling papers. I also did what I considered to be of major importance—teaching medical students the art of physical diagnosis.

We decided to take a trip to Europe and like everything else Trude did, if she was going to do it, she was going to do it right. She starting visiting travel agents and reading guide books, and before I knew it, had signed up for a six-week French course at the high school. I could still muddle through in German, but knew no French and she wanted to at least be able to ask directions, order food and buy things.

The package we chose was for twelve days in London and included tickets to shows in the West End, tours around the city and points of interest in the surrounding area and then a two-day visit to Paris. We thoroughly enjoyed London, and Trude especially liked the afternoon tea break, when she would pause to savor her favorite beverage and have a crumpet or two.

It was just a short flight from the Brighton Airport to Paris and then a bus took us to a small, quaint hotel in a neighborhood that was close to the opera, the underground, and a number of fine eating places such as Café de la Pais.

One of our first stops after seeing the monuments and the memorials was the Louvre. We spent most of an afternoon, oohing and ahhhing over the wonders of several centuries of art. Trude had specific pieces she wanted to see and had done her studying so was able to fill me in on the background of some of these great works. She also told me that the building itself was a fortress in the 13th century and as she kept telling me more of the history I found it interesting and really appreciated that she had done her homework.

Trude insisted we go to Montmarte, a short ride on the Metro from the Hotel Blackson where we were staying. Our first impression of the area was dramatic as we threaded our way up the steep streets and flights of steps leading to the famed Moulin Rouge in the nightclub district. The hill is crowned by the magnificent architectural mass of the Sacre Coeur Basilica, which gives the impression that Montmarte is topped by a sculpted cloud. The steps up the Basilica are mammoth, and inside the mosaics are beautiful beyond description. We climbed to the top of the dome and saw Paris spread out below us in all its grandeur. We were duly impressed and, of course Trude had her camera out quickly.

Squares of red paving bricks set in patterns formed the floor of the narrow, winding streets of Montmarte and two- and three-story houses in various color schemes lined the way, producing a delightful and happy feeling. Flowers in pots adorned the façade of almost every home. It seemed almost unreal, like a Hollywood set designer's conception of how Paris should look. Adjacent to this section was a block-square area swarming with artists selling their wares or offering their skills to paint any interested tourist. This was a real artist's colony. We learned later that such greats as Toulose Laetrec, Utrillo and van Gogh were part of the scene in years past, and now others had replaced them with hopes of being as renowned.

I looked for an artist who could do a charcoal study of Trude and one of me. A bust portrait would be fine. We found an artist but had to wait our turn, so we walked through the amazing display of every kind of artistic configuration imaginable, gaping and gawking and laughing and admiring what the artists were putting on canvas. Finally, Puette, one of the older, more experienced artists, drew Trude. She sat perfectly still as he delicately filled in the shading. He changed pencils and brushes rapidly as he went from her face to her hair to her clothes. The results were exceptional. Her facial expression was impressive and the portrait looked almost real.

After the artist was through, he asked Trude, "Parlez-vous fran-cais?"

She answered, "Je ne parle pas bien le francais."

He pointed to her completed portrait, "C'est tre's be."

She nodded, "Merci."

I said, "This picture belongs in the Louvre."

She smiled and said, "Oh, Zal."

I, too, had a sketch done. I looked grumpy.

We wandered about the district, stopping at various outdoor displays, or we'd find a small shop and browse the artists' works there. I was glad Trude had learned enough French so we would not be totally lost with the people we met. It proved very helpful even though our stay was brief.

As we walked along, passing shop after shop, a beautiful canvas displayed in a window of a very elegant store caught our attention and we went in.

"That would look so nice on the living room wall," she said, admiring the work. "We could hang it just over the spinet. It has so much depth and it's not too gaudy. But it's a little large to take back home. What do you think, Dear?"

I answered, "Yes, it's very nice, but how would we get it back? Maybe the store manager can send it to us. Let's ask."

She said, "I hope it's not too much, but everything here looks expensive. I'll ask."

She returned from talking to the clerk and said, "It's priced 750 francs. I don't think so. Too much money."

We looked further, and Trude spotted a portrait of the village of Montmarte. She was taken by it immediately, and said it was just what she wanted. It had clean lines in its perfectly contoured view of the street lined with red and white houses. In the distant background the two steeples of the Sacre Coeur peeked over the colorful rooftops. On one side of the street was a young woman, colorfully dressed in native garb, and on the other side, an older man wearing a cap and also looking very French. Next to him on an easel was a canvas, reflecting the twin steeples as in the larger drawing: a painting within a painting.

Trude studied the painting for a long time and then turned to me, "I wish I could do something like this."

"Maybe when we get home, you could take lessons again. And then you could have your own exhibit at one of those street fairs in Oak Park."

She smiled. We bought it and it hangs on the wall of our dining room next to the charcoal studies of Trude and me.

When we got back she did go to art classes at the Women's Club. I think her talent really came out in the use of charcoal and watercolors for the 12 pieces she finished. She even became quite good using oils. I wish she would have continued with her art since what she had done was quite remarkable and showed a use of symmetry and color that were appealing and appropriate. She got busy doing other things and eventually gave it up entirely. I think it may have also frustrated her that she could not immediately be spectacular at this as she was at so many other things such as French, investments, and music.

She had only taken piano lessons for a few years, but could still play beautifully. She would usually play show tunes, and often when I would see a book of music on sale I would buy it for her. Cole Porter tunes were her favorites, and one she learned to play quite well was "Wunderbar." I recorded the song on the tape recorder she bought me for Christmas one year, and that tape still makes for pleasant listening. Her rendition of "Tenderly" was so well done I tried to sing it each time she sat at the piano, but I think I detracted more than I added to her performance.

It had been fun to watch her and the children as they grew able to play more complicated musical pieces with greater ease. When Rick was at Yale, he played in a jazz band just for fun. We heard them play a few times, and the group sounded pretty good.

In 1975, Rick married a woman named Jodi Hack. She was also from the Chicago area, so luckily they were able to have a local wedding. She was a nurse and they seemed to hit it off quite well.

We took another trip to Europe in 1977, this time going to Yugoslavia. Unfortunately, we only had a few hours on our own away from the tour to try to find out a little of my family history or locate some relatives. With so little time and not knowing the language, I didn't make any progress. I did notice that each time I showed anyone my passport or had to give my name anywhere, the clerk or guard would smile and react to the name Zalar. Since I didn't know what they were saying but they were smiling, I could only assume that they were pleased to see someone from America visiting the old country.

Just for something different, we celebrated our 34th anniversary on Catalina Island off the coast of Southern California. Then we came back to the mainland and spent a night on the Queen Mary in Long Beach, where the ocean liner is a floating hotel. Of course we had a nice visit with Rick and Jodi while we were there. He was practicing medicine in Palos Verdes and delivering the babies of movie stars and sports figures.

Later that same year, I received a surprise phone call from a doctor friend, Clyde Kirchhoff, who was living in Ventura, just north of Los Angeles. Trude and I had visited him and his wife a year earlier on our trip to the coast. At the time, he invited us to see the group-practice clinic of which he had been a part for 22 years. He called to tell me that they need another specialist in internal medicine at their clinic and wanted to know if I might be interested in joining him and his colleagues. I told him I'd talk it over with Trude. Clyde and I were roommates in medical school, and we had kept in touch after we left the Army Medical Corps in '47. I thought it might be fun with the kids gone, and I guess we hit the empty-nest syndrome or mid-life malaise, and California sounded like a fun and exciting change.

After a few weeks of looking at all of the pros and the cons of such an adventurous shake-up in our staid but active life, the moving van pulled up to our home in River Forest. One factor that played a major part in the decision was that Rick and Jodi would be just about an hour's drive from us.

We had a great time enjoying our new surroundings. Most of our fun came from traveling to the various scenic spots in the state, and every weekend we were off someplace enjoying ourselves. We did all of the fun touristy things in the L.A. area including a trip to Burbank to see Johnny Carson on the "Tonight Show."

We also liked the music and theater scene in the area. Trude really liked Laguna in southern Orange County, with its many art galleries and resident artists. We still have a colorful portrait she saw and liked on one of our visits there. We enjoyed drives to the nearby desert or mountains, made a few trips to the wine country, and we visited Christian Brothers' Winery in northern California. Trude's father used to have his shot of their brandy each day and would live to be 91, so we went to pay tongue-in-cheek tribute to the good work of the good brothers.

While I was working at my practice, Trude busied herself at a hospital auxiliary and other volunteer jobs. When we weren't on the road, we had lots of visitors, and I would often come home from work to find friends or relatives lounging in the pool or in the lanai, sipping on a refreshing drink that Trude had concocted. Trude usually swam an hour a day in the large pool that came with our house— I can still see her doing her favorite side stroke. In the winter months, we would head for the ski slopes.

Although we liked many aspects of life in California, I didn't like the work at the clinic. I was seeing patients, but they were other doctors' patients, and I never really got to know any of them. I soon went looking for work and found it at the Kaiser Hospital in Hollywood. For nine months I worked as a medical consultant there, but the commute through L.A. traffic was no fun, so after some discussion, we moved back to our roots in the Chicago area, having stayed out West less than two years. In retrospect, I guess the move was a mistake, but it did shake things up a bit and make us appreciate life as it was. The grass is always greener.

Our daughter, Barbara Judy, had several friends who worked at Motorola, and she often would tag along on their ski-club outings even though she wasn't an employee. On one of these ski trips, she met a nice, young electrical engineer for the company, Ron Wesoloski, and after dating for a while, they got married. I proudly walked her down the aisle with her looking as radiant as Trude had 35 years earlier.

In 1979, we went back to Europe, this time with our friends Joe and Shirley Limacher. We took a cruise from Rotterdam down the Rhine into Germany, then drove around Germany to see more of the sights, including Munich, then drove across Switzerland.

Later that year, while visiting Judy back in Illinois, we received a call from Rick's wife in California, telling us he was in a hospital, having suffered a stroke while running a 10-kilometer race in Huntington Beach, not far from their home in Palos Verdes. He was only 32, and so we were besides ourselves with worry. We were on a plane and at his bedside in 12 hours. We stayed close by him until he was out of danger, then Trude stayed to help Jodi get him back on his feet. He was paralyzed on the right side of his body and was unable to speak for a while, but he made a full recovery and returned to his ob/gyn practice. Rick survived the ordeal, but sadly his marriage did not, and soon after he was well, they divorced.

I went back to St. Mary's in 1980, enticed by a nice salary and a new challenge as Chairman of the Department of Emergency Services and the newly-initiated helicopter program. I stayed with them until 1987, when I reached their retirement age of 65, then returned to private practice.

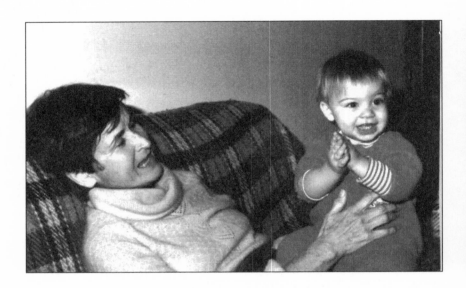

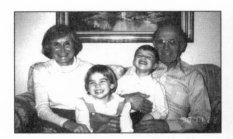

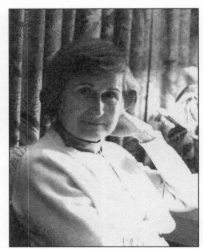

Trude and our grandson, Dave.
(top)

Trude and me with our laughing
grandchildren, Diana and Dave.

Trude looking thoughtful, 1983.

The Eighties and More

We continued traveling and in 1980 hit New Orleans for the first time—I was there for a medical conference, but as always with these medical trips, we managed to fit in some sightseeing. We had taken other such trips to other cities so that I could learn a few things, Trude could do some shopping, and we both could see the sights.

One of our trips in 1981 was to Denver to attend Judy's graduation. Ron and Judy (known to Ron and pretty much everyone else as Barbara) had moved to Colorado when Ron was offered a job out there. Ron and Barbara Judy bought a time share on the Texas coast and we were able to vacation there with them a few times.

Trude's father, Matt Pisut, Sr., died in 1981 at the age of 91. Sadly, when he passed there were few left who remembered all of the good work he had done in his community. Trude's sister Ag had always lived at home and after Trude's mother died in 1973, she took over the care of the house, her father and her sister Barbara. Ag put in long days, commuting to work in Chicago but coming home to Joliet each night to tend to the family. Barbara died in 1990, having lived an amazingly long time given her infirmities, and I am sure it was due to the excellent, loving care from her mother and sister. Ag died in 1995, having never married and having lived a very lonely life.

In 1982 we went to California to visit Rick and play a few rounds of golf, including a round at Pebble Beach. It's every bit as beautiful and tough a course as it appears to be on television, and at one point Rick hit a shot down to the beach. Having lost enough balls and taken enough penalty strokes, he decided to hike down to the beach and play his shot from the Pacific's large sand trap. As Trude and I stood by laughing, he played a beautiful shot back up onto the fairway—I think that may have been the only hole on which he came close to making par. When Trude would miss a shot, she would quietly say, "Damn." But if I missed a shot and swore, she would look at me and say, "Zal, please!" Of course, I was usually saying worse than "damn."

We also went to Florida shortly after the opening of Epcot. We had done Disneyland shortly after its opening years earlier so this seemed a nice thing to do. We played a little golf in Florida, too.

I had gotten in the habit of writing an annual Christmas letter and said in the one for 1983 that after getting checked out at the Mayo Clinic, we had "no remarkable problems," and that "some of our dear friends have not been so lucky." If only I knew then what was in store for us, I might not have been counting us so lucky.

As I got busier in my practice, Trude was getting interested in word processing and honing her secretarial skills with a thought to possibly going back to work. She had immensely enjoyed a word-processing course she had taken on the QE II on the way to Europe. We took a voyage on that luxury liner to England, docking in Southampton. The passenger list was full of notable names, but we commoners ate at a table with other nobodies from Philadelphia, Princeton and Cape Cod. We spent six days in London going to plays, including "Les Miserables," which Trude very much enjoyed. In Ireland, Trude wanted to kiss the Blarney Stone. To do so, she had to lie down on her back, and the attendant had to hold her arms so she didn't slip into the hole containing the stone. She arched her head back and kissed the famous piece of rock, laughing all the way. I did, too.

Trude's active mind required some stimulation, and I was so busy at work, one Christmas season she got a job in the linen department of the local Marshall Field's, more for something to do and not because we needed the money. She never got around to returning to work as a secretary.

On another vacation that year, to again try to explore how the other half lives, we took a trip to Mackinac Island in Michigan and stayed at the famous Grand Hotel. Trude and I liked the romantic setting and stately old lodging.

Many women seem to like to talk on the phone for hours, but Trude never did, and even when we lived far from our children, she wouldn't engage in lengthy phone chats with them, instead preferring to visit. The Olympics in Los Angeles in 1984 provided us with another excuse to go see Rick, and he went with us to the Opening Ceremonies and many of the athletic events that make the games so popular. It was truly a once-in-a-lifetime experience to see everyone from all over the world coming together, on their best behavior and being very polite. No one wanted us to walk away thinking that all Italians are rude or all Australians aren't fun, so the crowd was very well-behaved, and we had a good time chatting with people from so many countries and learning a little about them. We found the Games very different than when we had watched them on TV. At home all the announcers talked about was the medals race, but that seemed unimportant in the stadiums, where the international camaraderie was the main event.

Ron and Barbara Judy enjoyed the mountain living and skiing in Colorado, but Ron was happier at Motorola, so they returned to the Chicago area. Judy was very pregnant, and shortly after they got back, on October 15, 1984, she gave us our first grandchild, David Richard Wesoloski. They moved into our house in Barrington until their house was ready, and we moved into an apartment closer to my work. Trude and I planned to find a place that was more convenient for me and the apartment drastically shortened my commute, but when their house was done and they moved to Wheeling, northwest of Chicago, we moved back to our Barrington house because Trude missed the pool.

What Trude liked most about our house in California was being able to swim everyday, so we had a pool put in at our house in Barrington that was the same size as the one we had left out West.

Thanks to Dave's arrival on the scene, Trude now had something to do—play doting grandmother. She developed a special relationship with him and taught him patty-cake and other children's games. Perhaps because he was the first grandchild or because Judy needed more help with him, or thought she did because of her novice-parent status, Trude spent a lot of time with them. Trude may have remembered what it was like to be a first-time mother and how much she could have used help—which she didn't have—when Rick was born. The nice pool at the Barrington house made it possible for Judy, Dave, and Trude to swim together every afternoon that the weather permitted.

In a few years, Dave had a little sister, Diana Marie, born July 20, 1987. I enjoyed seeing the way Trude lit up around the grandkids. In our 1987 Christmas letter, I wrote that I was sure Dave, now three, loved her, but probably loved his Pinocchio film and trains better.

In our annual holiday letter to family and friends the next year, I lamented that as much as we enjoyed the grandchildren that it was a shame we were not 40 years younger so we could watch them grow up. I was reminded of the bumper sticker that said "If I'd have known grandchildren were so much fun, I would have had them first."

Trude got to spend a bit less time with Diana because we moved farther away and the drive across the city was not an easy one, so visits fell off to once a week or so. Also, her help was not needed as much since Barbara Judy was now an experienced mother.

We moved from Barrington back to Joliet in August, 1987. I guess as we got older, some sort of homing instinct had us wanting to return to our roots. The new yard was quite large and was enclosed with a high wooden fence. Trude busied herself applying her artistic talents to transforming the barren ground into a neighborhood showplace. Within a few weeks green sprouts were brightening the landscape.

When the proper time arrived, she transplanted each sprig individually and nourished them as though they were her children. In time, every color was present in the rainbow of zinnias she had planted. They all stood proud and tall, running the entire length of the fence for 50 feet, and she kept them watered and thriving into the autumn. It was amazing how quickly she had transformed the yard into a botanical garden.

The drought of '88 made it tough to grow anything but crabgrass and weeds. If I could have sold the weeds, I would've been ranked in the Fortune 500. While I lost my battle with the lawn, Trude managed to raise another crop of beautiful zinnias to distract from everything else wilting around them.

In 1987 Rick had a skiing accident in which he broke his spine on a ski run in Utah. After his surgery, his mother spent 10 weeks with him in California, once again playing nurse and mother as needed. Rick soon went back at work, delivering 200–300 babies per year. Later that year, he got remarried after he re-met his wife, Paula, at a high school reunion. They were both divorced and started corresponding; one thing led to another and they are now happily married.

Back in Illinois, Trude once again supervised a redecorating job as she fixed up the house the way she wanted it and somehow managed to keep her sanity among all of the comings and goings of the plumbers, painters, roofers, electricians, paperhangers, et al.

In 1991, my sister Dolores died, leaving me the last survivor of my immediate family. We also lost Trude's siblings Matt, Ag and Ann, who died a very short time afterwards, making us both too aware of our mortality.

On a more pleasant note, I recorded in the Christmas letter that our grandson, Dave, had reached the age of slang, and Trude and I would return from visits to the Wesoloskis laughing that everything in David's life was now "awesome." Diana was growing into a cute tomboy, willing to take on any challenge, including her brother. We found them both quite entertaining and wished we could spend more time with them. Trying to get back and forth from their home north of Chicago to ours south of the city was often an ordeal. It's often said that in Illinois there are only two seasons: winter and construction.

I got reflective in that year's Christmas letter after having just read Stephen Hawking's book, *"A Brief History of Time."* He wrote "We find ourselves in a bewildering world. We want to make sense of what we see around us ..." We hope that someone will discover a complete theory and then "we would know the mind of God." Years later, I would have too much time and lots of reasons to ask much about much weightier issues, but at the time I wrote that my biggest question for God would have been, "Why haven't the Cubs won a World Series since 1908?"

My love of classical music and operas had slowly seeped into Trude over the years, and we became rather regular patrons at the Civic Opera House in downtown Chicago. We also enjoyed the summer schedule of featured stars at a favorite haunt on the north shore of Chicago, a place called Ravinia. It was an outdoor venue, and along with friends, we'd eat our Saturday dinner on the lawn of the grounds just outside the pavilion. Also in attendance were a few hundred other music fans as well as some top entertainers such as Ella Fitzgerald, Tony Bennett, and the Chicago Symphony Orchestra, and the ambiance of the great outdoors made the programs complete. Trude always liked dining on the lawn, even though our table wasn't set with silver candlesticks as many of the others were.

Our last chance to attend a good musical performance was during a visit to Los Angeles in 1992. Rick got us tickets to a marvelous production, "The Phantom of the Opera."

The year previous, Barbara Judy had taken Dave and Diana to visit her brother in California, and the kids were able to play in the ocean and visit Mickey Mouse at Disneyland, as our kids had done when they were young.

By the end of the 1980s, Trude and I were in our late 60s and although we tried to do as much as we always did, that wasn't always possible. I knew I had more aches and pains than I used to and didn't notice any real changes in Trude, but I saw her every day, so any changes were too gradual for me to notice. For some people who had known Trude well, it was possible to see that she was not quite as sharp as she once was, mentally or physically. A little slowing is normal by that age, so if I had noticed anything, I wouldn't have taken it as a sign of what was coming. If I had, could I have done anything differently anyway?

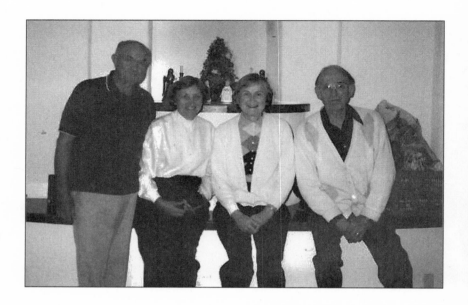

Trude and me with Tony and
Ginny Pantone (at left) Poway,
CA, 1992. (top)

Me and my old friend Bob
Gaspich.

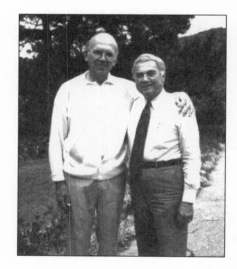

The Gathering Clouds

The trip to California in '92 seemed normal enough at the time: The visit with Rick and Paula was great, as was the Andrew Lloyd Webber musical. We took several more major trips that year, one that included a long drive from L.A. up the coast to visit our friends Bob and Marty Gaspich in Los Altos Hills, near the Silicon Valley. Only rich doctors and electronic whizzes could afford to live there: I don't qualify in the first category, but Bob did, and with my computer ignorance, I surely don't qualify for the second. We even made it all the way up to Seattle to visit a pediatrician friend, Bill Warrington, and his wife, Phyllis. We retraced our steps through Yosemite and a few of the other places we had gone so many years earlier with the kids.

We then headed back south to spend some time at Tony and Ginny Pantone's new house in Poway, California. We just kicked back and did nothing, although Ginny seemed to be on the go 23 hours a day. The Pantones had lived in Southern California for 14 years at this point, but we had known Tony since medical school and Army duty, and we had frequently visited back and forth over the years. In 1946, he had joined Trude and me as we traveled across the country from Chicago to my first Army assignment at Madigan General Hospital in Tacoma, Washington. We served as clinical physicians there until early 1947, when we were both transferred to Fort Lawton Station Hospital in Seattle, Washington, so these early years of medical and army life together had forged a pretty good bond that kept us rather close.

We stayed in this very pleasant area where the Pantones lived, about 25 miles north of San Diego. We had been guests at a resort complex there many years before, where we enjoyed playing golf, swimming, and other vacation fun. We also weren't too far from the ocean and took frequent trips to the beach.

Vivian Pironciak, who had been Trude's best friend and confidant when Trude and I were courting, lived in San Diego. She had never married and had moved to Southern California just after World War II. One day when our car was parked outside Viv's, our camera was stolen from the backseat of our car. We filed a police report, but of course it was never recovered, and I thought this was the only blot on what had otherwise been a perfect trip. It wasn't until after we were back home in Illinois that I realized something else had gone wrong.

When I first asked Trude to go steady a few months after we had met, she had agreed to wear my high school graduation ring and my fraternity pin, as was the tradition in those days. The next ring I gave her was an amethyst ring which I presented to her on her birthday in 1943. That was replaced about a year later with a diamond engagement ring, but at the time I couldn't afford anything expensive. When I bought it, I had sought the help of my brother-in-law, Fran Curry, who knew a jeweler in downtown Chicago—my sister Marion's husband seemed to have mysterious connections everywhere. He was the one who had hooked us up with hotel reservations and tickets for sold-out shows for our second honeymoon to New York in 1945. Some months before I had purchased that ring, Trude had been shopping in the Loop, where all the fashionable retail stores were located. In one of her letters, she wrote:

> Went by Lebolt's today and saw the most gorgeous diamond. Wow! Was it a whopper. It was 2.68 carats and the price was $1000.00. It had a sterling band, with 3 small diamonds on each side of the large stone. My boss has one similar to that; it's just beautiful.

She knew I couldn't afford anything like that, and she wore the one that I bought her proudly even though it was not very large—only one-quarter carat that cost $125, which was lot of money from my student wallet. Twenty three years later, I did go back to Lebolt's and buy one that was one and one-quarter carats, with one baguette diamond bordering the large stone on each side. It was almost flawless. Cost was much less of an issue this time and she wore it every chance she got.

Life settled down to our usual routine after our trip to California, and Trude seemed to have thoroughly enjoyed herself. One evening shortly after we were home, I heard Trude crying as I approached the bedroom. She was lying on her left side, and as I sat down next to her, I asked, "What's wrong, baby?"

She said, "I lost my diamond ring."

She couldn't remember when she had worn it last and I couldn't either. I thought she had it on while we were away, but she was too distraught to remember. Later when I thought back on this incident, I realized that although it would have been normal for her to be upset if she had lost her ring, her reaction was different than just being upset. If she had left it where we stayed in California, I could call and ask, but it was too late now. She didn't sleep well, and I stayed close to her throughout the long night. Something must have been going on inside of her that was nagging her. This was about a lot more than a lost ring.

In the morning, I called and spoke to the manager at the Bernardo Inn, where we had stayed. I asked to have the room searched, thinking Trude might have dropped it on the carpeted floor or left it in a drawer of the dresser, although I felt certain that if they had found it, they would have already contacted us. I even called the police to see if any jewelry might have somehow turned up. With the theft of the camera, I was wondering if the ring had somehow been stolen also. The search and inquiry turned up nothing.

I was sure the ring would never be recovered, so without telling Trude what I was up to, I drove to a jewelry store in Oak Brook near Joliet, where I had bought her other items over the years. After speaking to one of their experts, I ordered a new ring as close as possible to the one she had lost. Fortunately, I'd had all of the jewelry appraised recently and had a detailed description of each piece, including the missing diamond ring, so its features were almost duplicated. It took the jeweler about two weeks to get a copy. When I brought it home she seemed so pleased, smiling for the first time since she had noticed the other ring's absence.

A few days later I noticed Trude's red velvet jewelry case in the bedroom. I don't know why I had an urge to open it, as I had rarely done so over the years, but something told me to look. Upon releasing the lid from its lock, there, sparkling in the room's light, were not one diamond ring in the creased holder, but two! I called her to the bedroom and showed her what I'd found. She didn't seem happy or upset or surprised. I was happy, but shocked, since I hadn't thought to look in the box when she said the ring was lost. Her lack of reaction to the find baffled me as much as the discovery itself. Again, it wasn't until later that I realized just how unusual her reaction was.

Luckily, the 60-day time limit for returning the purchase hadn't expired, and I took the ring back to the store, much to the salesperson's dismay. That returned the money, but not my piece of mind as to why this happened in the first place—I would have gladly forgotten about the money if I could have known what this all meant. I was never sure how to raise the subject with her again, and after a while just let it drop.

I later asked Tony if he noticed anything unusual about Trude's behavior because it was on the vacation trip that the trouble had started, or at least that I first noticed something was wrong. As an old friend, Tony always felt comfortable being very blunt and to the point with me, and I'm sure he would've told me if anything seemed amiss to him, but it didn't.

Although there were little mishaps here and there, there was nothing else that really caught my attention, and we did some more traveling, including a trip to Boise in September, 1992, to see our old friends Ann and Dick Vycital. Dick was a classmate, and we had gone skiing with the Vycitals frequently over the years. Dick passed away a few months after we saw him, so I was glad we had this last chance to talk.

I tried to talk Trude into having the party for our 50th-wedding anniversary a year early so she could enjoy it. I couldn't bring myself to tell her what I feared, which was that by the following year she might be too far gone to even know what was going on. As shaky as her state now was, she was still clear-headed enough to make it known she wouldn't hear of having our party prematurely. At dinner one evening during the summer, I again made the suggestion of having a big party on our 49th anniversary instead of waiting for the 50th, and she replied very tersely and decisively, "I am not going."

When I asked her why not, she again said simply, "I am not going."

So we celebrated our 49th anniversary by going out to a nice restaurant with Russ and Jean Stevens, and Trude's sisters Agatha and Ann and Ann's husband, Jack. It was a quiet evening. For Christmas, we returned to California to spend it with Rick and Paula.

In retrospect I wonder what I was thinking, dragging Trude all over the country. Something clearly was not right, but I still tried to ignore it. The following spring, I had a medical conference to attend in Washington, D.C., so Trude and I drove there. She took in the sights while I went to seminars, and they had programs for the spouses as well. One of the pictures I saw after the trip bothered me. Trude, who usually sparkled even in a photo, looked completely blank and vacant, and more frequently, I had noticed her gazing off absently.

In 1993, I made an appointment for us both to be examined at the Mayo Clinic in Rochester, Minnesota, a six-hour drive from Joliet, where I had been myself two years earlier for a stomach problem. Before I set up the appointments, I talked to Trude about the need for her to have a physical examination. A silent problem with her heart, discovered years earlier, was due to be checked, even though she wasn't complaining of anything at this time. It was also about time to have her thyroid gland tested and be sure the treatment prescribed since 1987 was still controlling her metabolism properly.

She didn't know it, but as part of her doctor's visit, I had asked to have a neurologist see her. I was very worried about the changes in her normal way of doing things and her general mental state. It's not completely unknown for the thyroid gland or the medication that regulates it to cause behavioral changes. I knew it was a long shot, but still possible. My personal knowledge of what tests were to be done was vague, and I had only read or heard of their meaning. They were classed as cognitive tests measuring one's memory and thinking, not tests of intelligence.

This screening, known as a Mini-Mental State Examination, isn't anywhere near as complicated as an IQ test, SAT or GRE. There were very simple questions to test the patient's ability to recall, such as:

What are the year, the season, the date, the day, and the month?

Name three common objects, such as as penny, apple, table.

Name as many animals as you can in a minute. Eighteen is normal. Below 12 is cause for concern.

Count backwards from 100, by subtracting 7. This one may sound a little tricky at first, but for someone whose mind is functioning, even non-math oriented people, it shouldn't be that difficult, and obviously being off by a number or two was not crucial. 93, 86, 79, etc. Not being able to even attempt the task, or being off by tens, was a concern.

Mark the face of a clock with the correct time. Draw the outline of a house. Draw a flower. A kindergartener would be able to do these last few. Not great art, but in a way that any adult would be able to tell what the objects were supposed to be.

I sat in the busy reception room of the General Medicine Clinic, waiting for what seemed to be an interminably long time. I thought something had gone wrong. The door finally opened, and I went to meet her as she left the doctor's office. She had been crying. As soon as I reached her, she said, "I want to go home."

She was scheduled to have a consultation the following morning with the chairman of the Department of Neurology, but Trude was so quietly adamant in her desire to go that I told the secretary we were leaving.

During the long drive home, her eyes were never dry. We stopped only once to get a bite to eat at a drive-in, but she remained visibly shaken. Clearly Trude knew the tests hadn't gone at all well and was afraid of what that must mean.

Her examining doctor wrote to me a few days later to give me his findings. I had read many medical reports in my career, but none that cause me so much dread.

It was my pleasure to perform the history and physical examination for your wife during your recent visit to Rochester and she was also seen in consultation by Dr. O'Duffy, a fellow in advanced training. However, I see from her note that you were unable to stay to see Dr. Fealey of the Neurology staff. Dr. O'Duffy, on mental status examination noted decreased learning calculation construction and decreased memory and general fund of knowledge. She noted a marked language dysfunction and errors in speech. She felt that this likely represents a degenerative dementia probably of the Alzheimer's type with language function being the most prominent abnormality.

Dr. Paul Grieff

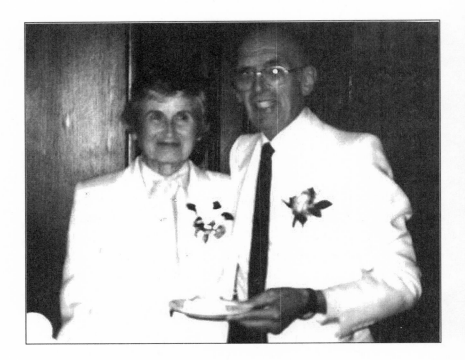

Trude and me at our 50th wedding anniversary party.

Trude's beloved Oldsmobile.

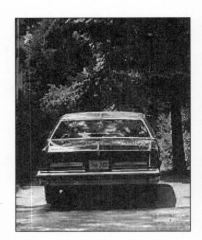

The Darkness Grows

As soon as I could compose myself enough to use the phone, I called the Mayo Clinic and asked for the specifics of Trude's test results. A secretary was kind enough to call me back after she had pulled Trude's chart and told me that Trude was able to score only 28 on the tests, whose normal score is 38. The smaller the score, the more the likely it is that there's a large amount of damage to the brain cells and their vital connections.

I wrote a letter to Rick in California:

Rick:

I am contemplating starting your mother on medication to see if there might be any chance of slowing down her gradual loss of certain nerve cells and the effect on her daily life. The newspapers are filled with info on the drug, Cognex (Tacrine). If you get a chance look for it in the trades and see what you think. Theory for use is acetylcholine and cholinergic fibers. It would be a shot in the dark.

My concerns with the medication are the possible body reactions, like nausea and loss of balance, and the need for blood testing on a weekly basis for some time. Whether I could get her to take the pill is uncertain and I would hate to have her become sick to her stomach since she eats well now and goes along at her own pace.

She has reached the point where our conversational exchange is almost nil. And she realizes her problem partially. The other morning she cried when she couldn't make her thoughts known to me at the breakfast table. She said, "I can't express myself."

Big troubles lie ahead and I fear for the time when she cannot go to the store and shop. No one understands her and dealing with that will be her downfall. So far she is just making it.

I would suggest the next time we speak that you talk more with her than with me. How is she? What is she doing? Anything new? Words to stimulate her. She will try to talk in her own jargon and be patient with her. When I don't understand what is said, I have to beat around the bush. Her greatest feat and that takes forever, is adding up our assets which has been her task is going to be difficult. There are mistakes, but who cares, as along as she has something to do.

Otherwise, beyond her cooking which is becoming a task and reading, which is haphazard, there is not much. So the days go on to a lingering few, and I get more and more upset with her problem since we cannot do much to stop it; unless I take a chance with the drug I mentioned. Our golden years are going to be difficult.

You will notice I used another address as a return. If this letter was returned and she opened it, she opens all mail but rarely reads it, I can imagine the consequences. The Mayo Clinic adventure was enuf.

Love,

Mom and Pop

After further investigating the available drugs, I couldn't find any that seemed to make a big enough difference to be worth the risk with side effects. With her communication skills failing fast, I wasn't sure if she would be able to tell me if something was wrong.

It wasn't long after the Mayo visit that Trude and I were just about finished with dinner when she placed her fork on the plate and looked straight at me, sort of like a plea for help, and said, "I can't remember anymore."

I didn't know what to say or how to answer her, but I tried to reassure her that everything would be okay. I'm sure that didn't help much, as I didn't believe it myself. She looked very scared and her eyes stared, silently pleading: Why? What's wrong with me? She left the table, and I waited a moment to steady myself, then walked into the family room, where she sat in her lounge chair. I knelt at her side and wiped the tear from her cheek and asked her if she would like to lie down on the sofa. She said nothing. She didn't answer my quiet assurances, and they seemed rather weak, even to me. What could I say when I knew better than she did that I didn't have the answer? I fell into silence and just stroked her hand. I got little sleep that night as I tried to think of what to do.

Deciding that 47 years was long enough, I left my practice. I had planned to retire soon anyway, and we were hoping to spend more time with family and friends. For some reason, in spite of the Mayo warning, I was thinking she might just be getting a little forgetful. At our age, who wasn't?

In July we took a trip to Des Moines for the wedding of our niece Gina Pisut, the daughter of Trude's youngest brother, Emery, and his wife, Rae. Trude seemed fine on this trip, a little more quiet then her usual subdued self, but certainly nothing to be remarked upon by any of the relatives we saw there, so in September, we headed back to California to see Rick again, and then headed north up the coast, then back down to Rancho Bernardo. It seems crazy in retrospect to have been running around like this with Trude having her spells now and then. Perhaps on some subconscious level I was trying to run away from our problems. If Trude was having problems, she largely kept them to herself. Sad to say, like many couples who have been married a very long time, we had almost run out of things to say. Or at least Trude had. As friends say, I can be a bit verbose and could carry on a conversation even if no one was listening.

Until June 1993, I was still in practice and I was gone from early morning until early evening. When I got home for dinner we ate with the TV on and spoke about the usual things, nothing too difficult. I always ate too fast while she chewed every morsel patiently silently listening as I prattled on about whatever. Trude was never a big talker, but when she said something I didn't notice any remarkable confusion or speaking difficulty. She was always sort of quiet and now was just a little more so. She continued to do the shopping, buy her own clothes and lead pretty much a normal life. At times I reminded myself of the Mayo diagnosis, and as I listened to Trude and observed her, I was sure they had to be wrong.

In June, 1994, we again visited Rick and Paula in California. Rick noticed that his mother was not nearly as clear-headed as she had been even on the last trip, but we didn't dwell on the topic.

Over the summer she seemer to go downhill fast, but I was so busy planning our anniversary party, I guess I was not paying nearly as much attention as I should have. I had arranged the whole thing by myself, and when I would ask Trude about the plans she would just say "Yes" or "No" without much elaboration.

The golden anniversary party was held at the Drury Lane Theater in Oakbrook, Illinois, on September 17, 1994. We held it one day late to make it easier for people who had to travel to get there. About 100 guests attended, some coming from as far away as Wisconsin, Nebraska, Florida, Ohio and California. My niece, Mary Alice Carney, who had been our flower girl, came from Texas with her husband and son. It was nice that so many friends and family would make so much effort to be here for us. Seven of the original eight members of the wedding party were still alive, and all but one were able to attend.

Trude spoke little, usually just nodding agreement with anything that was said—like the polite acknowledgement you give to a stranger on an airplane to whom you're not really listening.

I hired a videographer to tape the whole affair, and a microphone was passed around so everyone could say a little something. The comments of my longtime friend, Tony Malone, who was dying of cancer at this time, stand out: "You cannot imagine two finer people. They brought out the best in each other."

Our grandson, David, then 10 years old, was on crutches at the party as the result of a leg badly broken in horsing around with friends. On the video he shows up in the background hobbling around.

Trude was not well. I could see it, but I don't know how many others noticed. She would smile vacantly and say "Yes" or "Really?" or "thank you" or laugh at some of the jokes, but at other times just stared into space, seemingly unaware of what was going on. Some of the guests might have thought she just had the flu or was under the weather, and few would have guessed just how little Trude was comprehending.

My old friend Bob Gaspich stood up to tell the story of how instrumental he was in my meeting Trude, of when I had seen her photo in the newspaper and had asked him to go by Trude's office and check her out for me. Neither Bob nor I will ever forget his reply: "If you don't date her, I will." After telling this story, he added, "If I hadn't made the right decision, none of you would be here!" This got a big laugh from everyone but Trude, who was just staring with a smile frozen on her face, seemingly unaware that this story somehow concerned her.

As I thanked the assembled friends and family for their love over the years, I broke down and cried. As rapidly as she was worsening, I was much more aware than anyone there that this would be the last time Trude would see most of them, or at least would be cognizant of seeing them. Given the age of most of our friends, I guess it's not surprising that in the years since that party all but two of our siblings and probably half of our friends who attended have died.

In watching the video, I realized I sort of hogged the limelight but, of course, I always liked being the center of attention, and Trude did not. At any party or get-together, she usually let me do all of the talking, but I was struck by how little she shows up in this record of her 50th-anniversary party. I told my friend Russ Stevens that I felt bad and that it almost looked like I was ignoring her, but Russ said, "She was so sick then, you didn't want to embarrass her. She might not have known what to say, or been able to say anything." Maybe Russ was right, but when I watch that video, I still think I should have included her more.

Even a month after the party, she was worse. As the year dragged on, she was going downhill so fast, but it took a rather major event to wake me up to the fact that something was more than a little wrong.

On a rather cold and overcast day in November, Trude had gone to the neighborhood store to do her usual weekly shopping around 10 a.m. As the morning wore on I didn't pay attention to the time, since I was busy with the appliance repairman who had come to fix the dishwasher. After he left, I realized it was now after noon, and Trude still hadn't returned. Often her list of errands took a while, but I was sure she'd have told me if she weren't coming home for lunch. I couldn't imagine her having car problems so close to home, and if she had, she'd have certainly called.

Suddenly, the door from the garage into the house opened. There she was, a picture of fatigue and fright, carrying two full bags of groceries. Her face was drawn, and she was obviously cold. She was still, and her cheeks were red from the cold and the wind. She was staring blankly, and her hair was messed. I helped her take off her London Fog trench coat, which was certainly inadequate for a seven-block-long walk on a cold day, and as I helped her lie down on the couch, I asked where she had been.

She said, "The car was stolen. I walked home when I couldn't find it. It was gone."

I asked, "Why didn't you call me?"

"I couldn't find the phone number."

This answer puzzled me. I tried to let it pass while I comforted her.

I asked her to rest for a few minutes and said I would try to find out about the car. She treasured her maroon 1978 Regency Oldsmobile and cared for it dearly. She wouldn't hear of me buying her a new one even though this one was over 10 years old and had more than 120,000 miles on it. Almost every week, weather permitting, she would back the car out of the garage and wash it. After the car was dry and she had polished the finish, she would vacuum the rugs, wipe off the instrument panel and finally clean the windows until everything glistened. She kept watch as to when it needed an oil change or other maintenance to keep it running like new. She was so happy with the car that years earlier I had ordered vanity plates for her that read TRUDYZ.

After I was sure she was all right, I bundled up and walked to the store. As I neared the shopping mall, I grew tired just from the distance, and I found it hard to believe she had carried those two heavy bags this far in the cold.

Her car stood out blatantly in the rather small lot, which was not even half full. I had lost my car in a large lot before, as most people have, but I stood puzzling over how she could not have seen it here. And even more disturbing was her comment that she couldn't find the phone number to call home.

I returned the car to the garage at home. In my absence, Trude had realized that her glasses were also missing, and she had no idea where she had left them. I checked her purse and around where she was lying and they were nowhere to be seen. I retraced my steps to the store, and, amazingly, found them just off the sidewalk on a grassy area about a block from the shopping center. I had no idea how she had managed to drop them there.

She was still upset. I was afraid this drama, along with the exertion in the cold, would bring on another heart spell since she'd had an attack a few years earlier. I checked her pulse and blood pressure, which seemed okay, but she still seemed cold, as though something besides the temperature was chilling her to the bone. She spent the rest of the afternoon quietly resting under a blanket on the couch.

She never drove again.

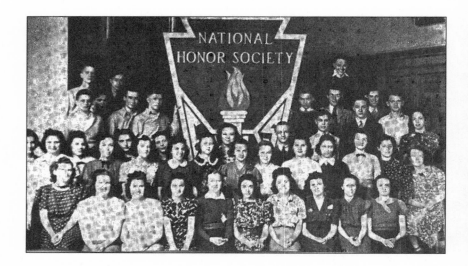

Our high school Honor Society photo. Trude is in the second row, fifth from the right. I am behind her and to the right. Garland McCowan, who helped Trude and I meet, is in the last row, farthest right.

Our friends in California, Bette and Gil McGirr.

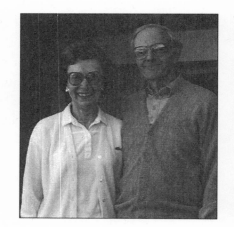

For Better or Worse

There was now no denying things would never be the same. I needed to spend more time looking after her and was almost afraid to leave her alone. She was getting worse daily, and I found myself having to help her with simple tasks. I didn't want to leave her by herself in the kitchen around the stove and other potential hazards. I had to double-check to make sure that this woman who took so much pride in her appearance went out properly dressed.

I had to think of what to do. I knew almost nothing about caring for an Alzheimer's patient and decided that I should move someplace where there were trained caregivers to see to her needs.

After checking around, I decided on an assisted-care facility in Rancho Bernardo, California, called the Remington Club. A friend had told me about it and said it was well-recommended as a quality place for seniors to live. It wasn't far from the Rancho Bernardo Inn where we had stayed a year and a half and a lifetime ago. Leaving our home on Buell Avenue in Joliet where our friends and our daughter and her family were fairly steady visitors wasn't easy, but I had to do something to help Trude make it through a day. After careful consideration, I bought a three-bedroom condominium just a short drive from the Club so it wouldn't be a chore to visit her, which I planned to everyday.

Rick and Paula still lived in Palos Verdes and were close enough that we were able to see each other quite often. It wasn't too much later that Rick retired for health reasons. In 2000, he and Paula moved to the rural community of Fallbrook, north of San Diego, to live quietly with their cats and dogs, so Paula could write.

In the past when we moved to a new home, Trude was the one who set everything up and dealt with the moving company beforehand. She took care of all of the details and watched over the whole process, correcting anything that wasn't as she wanted it. She usually kept me busy elsewhere, like the garage, the basement, or the attic, to be out of the way. There were joint decisions to be made as to what to keep and what to give away or sell, but somehow we'd get it all together. Now I had to do all of the work and make all of the decisions myself. As I dealt with the movers, utility companies and the rest, I started appreciating Trude's patience in having handled all of this without losing her sense of humor.

After the last box had been transferred from the moving van to the new condo, my job really began. It was a lot of work trying to decide what dish or vase or photo went where, and I found myself asking what Trude would have wanted or where she would have placed things. I just had to hope it was correct since she wasn't there to guide me. The biggest job was to empty all of the dozens of moving van containers, but luckily I had help from two friends who lived in the area, Gil and Betty McGirr. Gil's mother had died of Alzheimer's some years before, and his dad struggled to keep her well.

The one box I opened in the unpacking surprised and delighted me. It was the box in which Trude had saved all of our love letters: It was a time capsule not only of our lives including the 347 letters we exchanged during our courtship, but of what life was like in those days, when things seemed so much simpler. There were Christmas and birthday cards she had sent to me and then saved. After her French class, she had taken to signing many of them with such romantic tidbits as *To Mon Ami, Joyeux Noel-from Vous Ami* or *Votre Femme.*

I found my National Honor Society Certificate, which I had forgotten even existed. And I found her certificate as well. She had never told me she was in the Honor Society. Strange, but we were so busy living our lives we had never talked about such trivial details, and now it was too late. When I got out our yearbook from the Class of 1939, I found the photograph of the Society that showed Trude standing just below me. It seemed strange that I could have become so close to her over the years and stood that close to her then, and never said a word to her.

The suit box included her photo album from the 1930s and 1940s. She had all the cutely posed snapshots so popular then: some girls on swings in a park, another group on a merry-go-round; her father as a young businessman in a three-piece suit; Trude posing with another friend in their Sunday best and wearing hats. Another very cute photograph was of Trude and her dearest friend, Vivian Pironciak. Another photo showed Trude beaming her dazzling smile as she proudly stood in her cap and gown on the steps of JTHS.

She must have had lots of friends, since there were many snapshots of groups of girls and boys from the class and her autograph album was filled with good wishes and cute poems from those classmates. Near the end of the album were family photographs with her father and her brother Clement at age 5; her mother and her older sister, Agatha, dressed for church, and one of Trude in an evening gown, multicolored with a low neckline and a single white flower in her hair. Some of the most exciting for me were the poses in her bathing suit showing off her figure and her long shapely legs.

Finding the box was like finding part of her, but was made more painful by the fact that I couldn't sort through each piece with her and talk about the memories it brought back. She had no memories.

I don't know why she never told me she had saved all of this and had kept this box as her little secret, but I treasured all of these items now. With Trude becoming more and more absent, I found myself caught up in nostalgia, and looking through our letters brought back so many memories. Many times during the days and nights of her illness, I wondered if over the years of our marriage, Trude ever came to this cache of letters she had boxed from wherever they were stored in the house, took one at random, curled herself up in the lounge chair on a chilly winter night in the family room awaiting my return from my office, and read bits and pieces with a smile on her face and a feeling of warmth inside. If she did, she never told me. Why? I don't know, but I still wonder.

I have them all filed away in labeled boxes in our bedroom to keep them safe for Rick, and Judy and for her children, David and Diana, to look at when they are grown. Someday, in their eyes and thoughts, Trude and I will be able to live together again, but the contents can't possibly have the same emotional impact for the kids that those things did for me when I opened that box.

After we started having kids we were so busy living our lives that we didn't document it nearly as carefully and certainly didn't write each other long letters detailing our every activity. I wished now that we had.

Before we moved west, I had spoken to the Admissions Director of the Remington Club and others on the staff to arrange for a private room and the amenities to make Trude's stay as comfortable as could be, although I still felt a bit guilty about turning her over to the care of strangers. I was also feeling sorry for myself because for the first time in over 50 years I would be alone.

In order to assist anyone who would be part of her daily activities, I typed up Trude's daily routine which I thought might be helpful:

She gets up at 7 o'clock in the morning by an alarm clock.

She will try to brush her teeth each morning and night but someone is needed to place paste on her brush. Once in a while she may spread paste on her finger and use that technique.

She would forget to wash every morning and that was most unusual for a woman as meticulous as one can imagine prior to this illness.

I helped to wash her hair on Saturday. If it would be possible I would have the beautician do it while Trude is at the club and fix her hair so she looks nice.

I would put her clothes out and I would ask her if this or that is okay to wear. Socks were changed daily and I put the next day's pair on her shoes so she will not forget. The same pertains with her under-garments. I tried to place a new bra and panties or a panty girdle with her next day clothes but she has worn the same set if I didn't change them myself. I don't argue with her.

She sits at the vanity table fixing her face each morning but I don't have the slightest notion what she is applying and why. She has done this all her married life.

She eats almost all foods but she may try to cut mashed potatoes with her knife or when I was with her at the table, she will wait and see what I do with my dinner silverware. Assistance may be necessary but only on occasions. Sometime her dining habits are not the best and I do not correct them, realizing her control over what takes place is not as she would normally do it.

After our evening meal it was usual to go to the family room and read the papers and/or watch television. It was a diversion as it is for anyone, but now, the written word is lost and her appreciation for what is on the screen is not there. She does react to me when I talk, and there are momentary lapses into confusion. There seems to be little understanding. She likes movies and situation comedies on television but almost always, her interest fades and she falls asleep. And she may sleep on and off for two hours. Then all of a sudden, she is off to bed. She brushes her teeth, may take care of her face, and that's it. On occasions she will fail to take off her brassiere and her panties.

Our days were not very rewarding. She had a fixation on her purse, constantly arranging and rearranging it. She asked questions I couldn't always answer and then she'd cry. I finally bridged the problem by doing something else or changing the subject.

It looked as if she was adjusting to this new home, but that didn't last very long. When we were together she seemed fine, but I felt so sorry for her when I left, and she looked for me continuously, waiting at the front door of the building for my return. I spent as much time as I could with her, including eating our meals together in the dining room, and she seemed to be content, but after I would say goodnight and leave, she would act up. I learned that this was common with Alzheimer's patients and was known as "sundowning." There was something about dusk that frightened many of them and was even known to cause violence in some people. Whether Trude's agitation each evening was due to my departure or sundowning or some other reason, I don't know.

Of her first 20 days there, she was alone only three, and I was told that during my absences she paced the floors and at times would wait by the front entrance to the club as though expecting my return.

When I arrived one morning, her clothes were strewn over the floor of her room, and she was lying in her bed not saying a word. None of the staff offered any sort of explanation, and of course Trude wasn't able to communicate one. Another time, I noticed the antenna on the television set lay on a table, broken off. This incident didn't cause any concern to the nursing assistants, but it frightened me. Since I was still unaware of all of the manifestations of this disease, I didn't know if she might need a medical examination or if some form of treatment could lessen her aggressiveness. The other residents seemed to be living more calm and sedate lives as far as I could tell, but I don't think my long list of concerns managed to make much of an impression on the admissions director.

Once I thought Trude was settled, although I wasn't sure how happily or quietly, I had to go back to Joliet to take care of a few matters. I wouldn't be gone long, at most four days. So that Trude wouldn't be left completely alone in unfamiliar surroundings, I had arranged for her oldest sister, Agatha, to come to California to be with her during the daytime hours while I was away. Once again, Ag was called upon to look after her family; I felt bad having to impose upon her, but also knew that she would be happy to help—looking after others was what she did.

I called the nursing coordinator at the Club daily to be sure Trude was all right, but one evening when I phoned I was told of an incident with Trude that frightened me terribly. They said she tried to stick the end of a paper clip into a wall socket. After that bizarre event, she was watched carefully until I arrived, and I changed my plans to return immediately. Clearly they and I had misjudged just how dangerous her dementia was becoming. During the flight on the plane, I thought of the possibility of Trude being seriously injured or even electrocuted. I read later that this sort of behavior was not uncommon at certain stages of Alzheimer's and that trying to stick things in electrical outlets was far from a rare occurrence.

She was quickly sliding into more severe phases of the disease, and no one seemed to have any good ideas as to what could be done. As a doctor, I was used to treating things, or at least seeing a clear progression of symptoms during the course of an illness. But now it seemed anything was possible in no set pattern, and worst of all, there was no way to even alleviate the symptoms, let alone treat the disease.

I arrived in San Diego at 6 a.m. and immediately went to the Club. She was alone in her room, and she wasn't herself at all, saying very little. I'm sure she felt I had deserted her. I went to her as she lay in bed and kissed her. Touching her hand and holding it in mine, I said, "Hi, Baby Dear. I'm sure glad I'm back. I missed you so much and worried how you were doing. I had to fly to Joliet. The deal for the house was done quickly after I signed the papers for us. I didn't get a chance to see or talk to Ag, but she knew I was returning today. I'll get everything packed up, and we're going back to the condominium. You'll like it. And then, after lunch, we can go to Escondido and look around. Okay?" She nodded yes. I thought she was going to cry, and me with her.

I learned that an assisted-living environment is just what the term implies. Each patient is expected to take care of herself with the help of a staff member, if necessary. Trude was no longer capable of even partially caring for herself or of being left alone when staff only made rounds at irregular intervals.

I didn't think they were doing a very good job looking after her and thought I could do better . I reasoned that if I was going to have to personally keep an eye on her 24 hours a day, I might as well do that at home. I moved her out of the Club and into the condo.

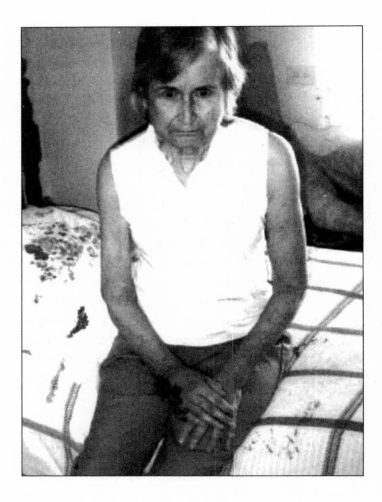

Trude lost in the disease.

This Damned Disease

One aspect of Alzheimer's that has been noted by many neurologists is denial on the part of the family. The people closest to a patient often refuse to accept what is happening to their loved one and want to keep thinking things will somehow get better. I was as guilty of this as anyone and didn't want to believe my dear Trude could really be losing her mind. If she was never going to come back to who she was, I was also having a very hard time accepting that she was getting worse. But after seeing that even a care facility was unable to handle her, and that it might not be safe for either one of us with her at home, there was now no denying it. I had to face the fact that what I had been reading about the disease—the whole disturbing picture—was coming into focus with Trude.

At first I was stunned that I could be so ignorant of a disease as prevalent as this one, but when I thought back to my medical practice, I realized I'd had no regular contact with patients who suffered from dementia. My first assignment in the Army was treating soldiers who ranged from mildly mentally ill to completely psychotic, but none who suffered from this sort of dementia. Occasionally in my years of family practice, I would be consulted by someone whose mother was getting forgetful, or whose father was getting lost, but I had never observed anyone on a daily basis as their faculties diminished. When I was called to a nursing home to attend to patients, my concern was their physical ailments, not their mental states.

If I ever had the chance to meet Dr. Alois Alzheimer, part of me would want to thank him for being so astute as to have so accurately cataloged this malady, and part of me would want to castigate him for having so accurately foretold the terrible future that awaited my Trude. I soon found myself wanting to learn all I could about the disease, including its history.

Alois Alzheimer began his medical career in 1888 in Germany and specialized in diseases of the nervous system. He spent more than a decade collecting data on patients with syphilis, its effects on the brain, and the symptoms produced. His skills in pathology made it possible for him to find and see the cause in the laboratory or under the microscope, and so to see the end result of a disease process. Then, in 1901 he started to take care of a patient known in the medical literature as simply "Auguste D."

In his notes, he told of her dramatic behavioral changes, memory loss, anxiousness, wild imagination, hallucinations, and inability to tell time. She died in 1906, as she had just reached her 56th birthday. She was considered psychotic because of her strange behavior, but when he performed an autopsy he found changes in her brain tissues. If anyone had recognized similar abnormalities before, they had never let it be known, and it wasn't until long after Dr. Alzheimer died that the full implication of his findings became apparent. Only a few decades ago his report was found hidden in the archives in a medical library and publicized as the important discovery it was.

He never fully appreciated what he had described in detail, and would almost certainly be surprised to find that the disease which bears his name is reaching epidemic proportions today and threatens to overwhelm our health-care system and our economy's ability to cope with the growing number of patients. As medical advances make it possible for people to routinely live to be 80 or 90, the population of Alzheimer's patients and potential patients is multiplying.

At the turn of the 20th century, Alois Alzheimer was asked what he might someday be remembered for, if anything, and he said something to the effect of, "For my knowledge of the disease syphilis as it affects the brain." He had been a pioneer in the study of that disease and had become known for his expertise in epilepsy and birth control also, but it was his work with Auguste D. that would make his name a household word posthumously and his childhood home in Marktbreit, Germany, a museum.

In 1910, a colleague of his wrote in a book of psychiatry: "The clinical interpretation of this Alzhemer's disease is still unclear. We are dealing with a serious form of senile dementia and the fact remains this disease sometimes starts as early as the late forties."

In all of my research, I found it very disappointing that almost 100 years later we know little more than Dr. Alzheimer did. With all the advances in diagnosis and treatment we aren't a lot closer to understanding the cause or treating this disease than the good doctor himself was. MRIs and other brain-scanning techniques have been helpful in screening for Alzheimer's, but even those fail to identify patients with complete accuracy.

Like weather forecasting, although the science has advanced greatly in the last few years, and there have been tremendous improvements in diagnostic equipment, we are still frequently wrong. And, as when we deal with weather, just because we know a tornado is coming, doesn't mean we can do anything to control the damage or change the outcome.

I knew it was rare for such strange behavior to be due to a thyroid problem, but since it can be so easily screened for, it is checked routinely before assuming Alzheimer's. Even metabolic imbalances, such as a magnesium or sodium level that is way off, could cause, in rare cases, some wild personality changes, but again, simple tests rule those out.

Creutzfeld-Jakob Disease, which is sort of the human equivalent of "Mad Cow Disease," also can manifest itself in symptoms that may mimic those of Alzheimer's, but a new test can reveal the cause. But it also moves much faster than Alzheimer's, and the patient is usually dead in 12–18 months. The dementia associated with Creutzfeld-Jakob was ascribed to a host of other things, including, sometimes, Alzheimer's.

Unlike so many diseases for which a simple blood or urine test can tell the tale, it's hard to treat a disease when it's impossible to be certain what the disease is. I found it frustrating that these doctors were willing to "guess" at a diagnosis. I was used to things being clear; a person had a disease or they didn't; you could treat it or you couldn't, but here was a brain disorder that may or may not be genetic and mysteriously appears without any flourish of fever, rash, or pain, and is untreatable. It seemed like sort of an inexact science to me to just rule out most other possibilities and then, as a last resort, hang a label of Alzheimer's on it. Its course is, was, and continues to be, unrelenting.

Neurological disorders are often only diagnosed by ruling out other causes, and then often the physician is left treating the symptoms since treating the disease isn't possible. Trude's diagnosis was a harsh refresher course in neurology for me and made me glad I specialized in internal medicine, where cause and effect were clearer.

I often read the statistic that 4 million Americans now have Alzheimer's disease, but that figure comes from a study that many experts now believe to be seriously flawed. Another study puts the number at 1.9 million in the U.S. which is probably more realistic, but again is based on just the percentage of the population that is a certain age and therefore likely to have the disease. No one has a real number of actual patients who have been diagnosed. Since it impossible to have a definitive diagnosis without an autopsy, it's difficult to come up with an accurate number. Whatever the number, it is large and steadily increasing—the risk of getting Alzheimer's disease just about doubles every five years after age 65.

One study showed that nearly half of people 85 and up have some form of dementia, but doctors are keen to point out that not everyone gets it and that senility or dementia are not just standard parts of aging, which was assumed to be the case for a long time. It was the relative youth of Auguste D. that made Dr. Alzheimer take particular notice of her symptoms.

It is normal to lose brain cells as one ages, but with Alzheimer's the cells and their vital connections are lost in large numbers—parts of the brain simply atrophy and stop functioning. With Trude, her physicians and I knew certain cells in her brain had stopped working, probably never to return to their normal use, but what cells were going to quit next and what this might mean in terms of her bodily functions or behavior—although doctors and books could try to give me some idea of what to expect—the disease still left a large range of unpredictability.

Before a patient dies, a diagnosis of Alzheimer's disease can only be made by the process of elimination and circumstantial evidence. Once the other possible causes of similar symptoms—strokes, tumors, viral and vascular diseases, and a variety of other maladies have been ruled out, it is said to be Alzheimer's. But, according to the latest data from the National Institute of Health, this is only accurate 90 percent of the time when compared with the actual results of autopsies. Since the majority of Alzheimer's patients are elderly and the majority of elderly people are not autopsied when they die, it's hard to get a firm grasp of the problem.

There are many causes of behavioral changes, but in the case of a head injury, for instance, the changes would be rapid, not the slow onset of Alzheimer's. Parkinson's disease, ALS (Lou Gehrig's disease), and multiple sclerosis all have rare forms that can sometimes mimic the dementia of Alzheimer's, but there are almost always symptoms of those diseases present before dementia sets in. Severe long-term alcoholism or use of certain drugs (both legal and illegal) can also be responsible for erratic behavior, but a patient history would quickly indicate the problem.

In Trude's case, we ruled out such causes, but I found myself still hoping that there could be some treatable problem. Even a brain tumor could have seemed a better of the bad possibilities that were now presenting themselves. At least there would have been some hope that after surgery she would be back to normal. None of the tests showed anything but what I feared, however—that she was going to slowly lose her mind to Alzheimer's.

I found much of my reading frustrating and discouraging. Not only was there no way to know for certain if Trude had the disease, but there was nothing to be done for her if she did. In his journal, Alois Alzheimer wrote of Auguste D. that her frequent answers to his questions was, "I have lost myself," and I could see and hear similar signs of frustration from Trude every day.

I found myself reading every mention of senility I could find. Shakespeare wrote about very old age as a time of "second childishness and mere oblivion."

In his book *Time Flies*, Bill Cosby joked, "Don't worry about senility, when it hits you, you won't know it." It is a glib, funny line, the kind for which Mr. Cosby is noted, but sadly, that's not true. Oblivion would be preferable to the knowledge that things were slipping away. Trude was aware, sometimes more than others, and often painfully so, that memories would never return, thoughts half-formed would never come into focus.

Like most people, I find it a little frustrating when I can't remember the name of a movie, who sang a certain song, where my car keys are or where I set my glasses, but such common glitches, which become more common with age, aren't cause for a panic attack, because I know I will remember. Even if I don't anytime soon, it's not the harbinger of impending doom.

With Trude, the frustration grew. Losing the names of even inconsequential things was annoying, and losing major things was the source of much pain and, often, anger. Even providing her with the forgotten item or name did nothing to stop the fear of the fog that was engulfing her. It has been stated that the rage of an Alzheimer's patient is neuro-pathological disease, and not just the emotional response to a problem like forgetting a word.

Carey Henderson, who was affected by Alzheimer's and kept a running diary of his thoughts and emotions as long as he was able, said with great accuracy, "With Alzheimer's people, there's no such thing as having a day which is like another day. Every day is separate .... It's as if every day you have never seen anything before like what you're seeing right now."

I don't think many people give much thought to their ability to remember things. A child's main concern is whether he will remember the facts long enough to spew them out on a test. During middle age, a person can become unhappy with himself for forgetting the name of a person he just met. Beyond the fifth decade, there is a tendency to become a little more upset as memory lapses seem to get more frequent. Past age 65, one never knows if this is just another lapse or the start of real cause for concern. For the most part, we seem to remember what we're supposed to know and forgot the trivia in our lives. Forgetting is normal and may be one of the brain's defense mechanisms against too much information or at least that's the premise that is sometimes offered. By 70 years of age, most people are showing a few signs of memory loss, but this is to be expected given the natural loss of brain cells. For some unknown reason, women usually seem to be less affected than men.

There are two different scales of Alzheimer's disease, one with seven stages and one with three. Like Fahrenheit and Celsius, they are just two ways of expressing the same thing, and whichever chart I consulted it was clear that Trude was racing toward the final stage: a mere shell, unable to do anything for herself. Once in this final stage, people have been known to live for years. According to the National Institutes of Health, most patients live 8 to 10 years after they are diagnosed, and living for 20 years or more in this sad state is not unusual. In the disease's later stages the patient often becomes bedridden, then dies of some other disease, perhaps a bladder infection or pneumonia, which is what kills the majority of Alzheimer's victims.

I felt as though I were lashed to the mast of a boat headed for the rocks and there was nothing I could do except watch the danger grow ever closer and curse my fate. I felt so powerless. All my reading failed to turn up any way to slow or stop this disaster from happening.

I often came upon Trude when she was crying—when part of her brain was functioning enough to recognize what was happening to the rest of her—the fear would overwhelm her. And I was often crying myself when I thought about just how hopeless the situation was.

Alzheimer's is not just advanced amnesia wherein a person forgets everything he ever learned, but parts of the brain actually atrophy and die so that bodily functions are no longer possible. The person may lose the ability to walk or speak or even to control or release their bowels. Medical science may now understand what happens—how plaque builds up in the brain, impeding certain functions, and how neurofibrillary tangles scramble messages like crossed telephone wires—but why it happens or what can be done to prevent it is still a mystery.

Early-onset Alzheimer's (hitting before age 65) seems to be most often genetic, that is, it runs in families. It also seems to progress faster than the late-onset variety. Cholesterol and plaque both seem to play a role in Alzheimer's, but one of the problems with finding the key to this disease is that there always seem to be too many exceptions to make any rule iron-clad. There seem to be correlations for some of these factors, and researchers are exploring many possible paths, but none has yet provided the one vital link, the way smoking does to emphysema. There are some studies that suggest that lowering the cholesterol in people with elevated levels may reduce their risk of Alzheimer's or that taking ibuprofen or vitamin E may also reduce one's chances, but so far nothing has been demonstrated to be a magic bullet or lay the groundwork for some sort of vaccine or antidote. It seemed every day I would read of some new promising lead, but nothing concrete that was going to make any large difference anytime soon.

I read one study that suggested that the smarter a person was, the less likely he or she was to get Alzheimer's disease, but I would take objection to that on a few counts, not the least of which is that Trude was brilliant. And certainly people more intelligent than she had gotten it as well, including the noted neurosurgeon Dr. John Douglas French, for whom an Alzheimer's-care facility in Los Alamitos, California, was named. The research that prompted the idea of an intelligence link was a study of nuns in which it was found that those who seemed brighter when they were younger, based on the scores of various tests they took when they entered the nunnery as teenagers, were apparently less likely to develop Alzheimer's.

Another neurologist I spoke to also took issue with this conclusion. Although he never did a scientific study to verify his observations, it seemed to him from his years of seeing patients in various stages of the disease that it wasn't that better-educated people didn't get the disease, just that they were smart enough to mask the symptoms longer. He theorized that better-educated people got the disease as often as less-educated people, but were able to use their advanced powers of expression to consciously or subconsciously mask the symptoms. If a woman could put off any outward signs of Alzheimer's for a few years, and then die of something else, no one may ever have known she had Alzheimer's. If a hypothetical patient were to develop Alzheimer's when she was 80, but was clever enough to not show it to anyone, and then died of heart disease at 83, no one was likely to perform an autopsy and remove the brain to see that there may have been severe brain damage. This neurologist saw one patient, a brilliant chemist who had been going to work every day and performing well, although he had not been able to write for two years because Alzheimer's had claimed that part of his brain. Although this Ph.D. could still express himself well orally, he had completely lost the ability to use abstract reasoning—which is one of the first functions to go with Alzheimer's.

Not only does the patient sense something is wrong and want to deny it, but a similar phenomenon takes place in the family, who see things were a little off but go into denial because they might not like the answers if they start asking questions. Just as the family of an alcoholic often works as hard as the alcoholic (sometimes consciously and sometimes unconsciously), to pretend there's not a problem, so too the reality of Alzheimer's is so painful that many avert their eyes rather than see the truth.

I had to admit afterwards that I was guilty of this. There were little signs, but I either was not paying enough attention, or didn't want to acknowledge what I was seeing. And again there is the other awful truth: even if I had known right away, it wasn't something like HIV or cancer, which if caught early is much more treatable than after the disease has reached fatal proportions in the body.

Another point about the intelligence factor is that intelligent people tend to do more, longer. Rather than be content watching reruns on TV, which is enough to dull anyone's ability to think clearly, people with higher IQs are more likely to want to go on traveling, learning, and doing things that keep their brains stimulated. In the nun study, the nuns who had higher scores when they were younger were often seen to go on teaching or working into their 80s or even their 90s.

John Bayley wrote in *Elegy for Iris*, his touching portrait of his wife, novelist Iris Murdoch, who died after a four-year slide into Alzheimer's oblivion: "… she was formidably learned." Clearly one of the most acclaimed British authors of the 20th century could not be placed at the lower end of the intelligence scale, yet she succumbed to the disease. Bayley's book was made into the movie, *Iris*, which helped bring the sadness of Alzheimer's home to a lot of people.

The awareness about Alzheimer's has increased phenomenally in the past few years, and that has led to an increase in research and care options. Just as Rock Hudson's death from AIDS put a face on that disease and made many people aware in a way they never had been and Michael J. Fox's battle with Parkinson's brought that into the public focus, Ronald Reagan and more recently, Charlton Heston, have put much-recognized faces on Alzheimer's. At times I wonder, as others have wondered about me—if Nancy Reagan is doing the former president any favors taking such good care of him that he continues in good physical health for so long after his mind was gone. I do believe it is very considerate of her to keep him out of the public eye so he can be remembered as he was, not as he is.

Knowing what was happening and even the clinical explanation of what was happening with plaque and connections in the brain did little to help me understand what was happening to Trude or what could be done about it.

As time wore on, other signs of Trude's disease were becoming more common. She was unable to select the correct clothing to wear and that was really difficult for her. An urge to take an already-made bed apart and remake it was becoming almost a daily ritual as were crying spells when she could not remember something. She often didn't seem to know what to do with food on her plate, or how to care for her personal bodily functions. It was like doing a picture puzzle in reverse, taking away pieces of her life and her normal function. As each piece disappeared, it had a frightening impact on her mental stability. Life's routines were simply coming apart. She often seemed terrified by her inability to know what to do and would stand frozen, trying to comprehend the maze her life had become. As I watched the abnormal become commonplace, I realized what the future had in store and wondered how I would cope.

I know the intense frustration on the part of anyone watching a loved one become lost, but perhaps I felt even more as a physician. I had learned much, but never did I have anything like Trude's continuing and worsening chain of mishaps to solve. With some illnesses it's possible to observe and do nothing—the disease will take its course and the best the doctor can do is ease the suffering. But with this, it was very hard to stand by and do nothing, especially when the suffering was of such an excruciating mental nature and there was no drug or procedure to ease the pain.

The dismal report from Dr. Grieff at the Mayo Clinic Medical center was becoming too real.

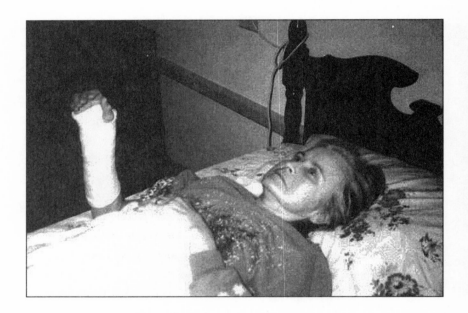

Trude with her broken arm

The Danger Grows

I began our Christmas letter for '95 with the observation that "if I had known what was to transpire since December 31, 1994, I would have stolen a line from an old musical, "Stop the World, I Want to Get Off." I went on to recap the year:

Rick was doing well and was widely recognized for his work in recognizing and preventing premature labor in expectant mothers.

Ron and Judy continue to do an excellent job with the kids: David is quite sharp and can talk anyone into anything and will probably end up president of something. He has a line so long and convincing you could, as Trude once wrote to me about her boss, "hang the Monday wash on it." Diana is smart and is already on her way somewhere.

I finished the two-hour video biography of Trude's life, and although I showed it to her, she is unable to appreciate what it is about.

I miss practicing medicine, although I still get occasional calls from patients. I liked the challenge it brought to my life and although I am still inundated with medical journals, filled with new and innovative approaches and hope for the future for treating, curing or preventing a variety of diseases, none of them offer any help for my own burden which gets heavier each day.

We didn't stay long in the condo. If I was going to have to care for Trude, I wanted to do it in familiar surroundings, and with the help of family, friends and medical facilities I trusted and where I was known. We moved back to our home on Buell Avenue in Joliet, but I knew we couldn't stay long since I had already sold the house and the new owners were to take possession in a few weeks.

Trude's level of sickness became alarming and bewildering. She showed personality changes and behavioral upsets like agitation, but not very often and nothing too severe until one evening about 9:30. I wanted to type a long-overdue reply to a friend's letter before going to bed. I was crossing the family room to go into the den when I saw Trude coming out of the kitchen right at me. There was something frightening about her, even before she got to me. Her eyes were wild and they seemed to bounce around independent of each other. Her lips were tightly pursed, as though she was about to explode. She flung herself at me, grabbing me and shaking me with all of her might—her whole demeanor was terrifying. I had the momentary thought that this was a scene from a bad movie where demons suddenly possessed the body of some innocent, mild-mannered person. But the violent shaking snapped me back to the harsh reality that my own wife was attacking me in my own house.

I tried to grab her and yelled, "Stop it! What are you doing?" She paid no heed whatsoever, which really worried me. There seemed to be no recognition of who I was, or that I was even saying anything, but I pleaded again, "Stop it! You're going to hurt me or yourself. Stop it!"

I grabbed her, and we half-wrestled across the family room toward the front door of the house. I tried grabbing her wrists, but her strength was amazing and she broke away from me and renewed the assault. She seemed to have no apparent objective, just trying to hurt me any way she could with haphazard pushing, pulling and grabbing. I didn't want to hurt her by fighting back too much, so I retreated toward the den. She was right behind me, shoving and pushing at me the whole time. Just as I reached the door to the room, she grabbed at me again, and I had to fight hard to break her grasp, pleading, "What is wrong? What are you doing? Stop this!" She said nothing, just continued in her silent fury until I wrenched her left hand free of me. She faltered backward, and I used this opportunity to slip into the den and close the door.

Getting free gave me a sense of relief, and I had a moment to catch my breath. After all, I was in my early 70s and not really in shape for the running battle I'd just had.

I fell into the desk chair and stared at the word processor, panting and dumbfounded by what had just happened. I could not imagine what had provoked this.

I was still looking for rational causes for manifestations of a disease that had no rational explanation. I sat there wondering if I had done something now or in the past that could have made her so insanely angry. I had read that such outbursts were not uncommon during some stages of Alzheimer's, but still had a hard time believing Trude could have sunk to this sort of werewolf behavior. Some patients are known to stay in this phase for years and have to be kept sedated or restrained. Some are set off by certain sounds, or bright lights, or just the coming of night. There are various theories offered as to why these fits occur—perhaps as memory fails she didn't recognize me and saw me as an intruder in her home who presented a danger to her; maybe she did remember some ancient grudge against me as though it just happened and wanted to settle the score. There was no way of knowing, and by the time people reach this stage, they are no longer capable of communicating clearly enough to offer many clues.

After I tried to calm down, I walked to the door and listened. It was quiet in the hall, and I opened the door carefully, peering out to see if she might be waiting for me.

She wasn't in the hall. I walked quietly to the family room, but she wasn't there either. The clock on the television now read 10:20. I walked softly through the room, toward our bedroom, turning out the lights along the way. She was in bed, sleeping laying on her left side, facing away from my pillow. I got undressed quietly and slipped into bed beside her.

I lay awake most of the night, partly out of fear and partly out of worry. Had the dementia turned violent? How long could this go on?

Had I lost her forever? She slept silently beside me, apparently not bothered by the evening's events.

The morning light came around the window shade and woke me. I knew I hadn't been asleep long. She was still and quiet beside me. I quietly rose to use the bathroom and when I came back I saw that she was awake, but something didn't seem quite right, so I was hesitant about speaking to her. I waited for her to move. About an hour later, she finally pushed back the covers to get up, but her movements told me something was wrong.

I could see immediately that she was in pain, and she stood, her right arm dangling uselessly at her side. She had tears in her eyes and seemed a little unsteady on her feet, so I quickly went to her and helped her sit back down on the edge of the bed.

I looked at her arm and saw the black-and-blue marks on her left wrist. My grasp of her arm was more than I realized at the time of our struggle last evening. I went to reach for her right forearm to look at that as well, but she moved away from me. She said nothing and she had a strange look in her eyes. I looked at her arm without touching it and could see there was a bulge at the inside of the wrist where it meets the hand and, even without touching it, could see that it appeared to be badly broken. I had seen enough broken bones over the years to know this didn't look right. When we were struggling with each other, she must have fallen backwards as I pushed away to escape into the den. She probably tried to use the right arm to break her fall. She must have suffered all night long in pain and never made a sound, but lately her speaking had been limited to a few words she used repeatedly—like "Yes" and "Really?" and often she used them without meaning, so it may have been impossible for her to tell me what was wrong.

I was quite angry with myself for not having noticed this last night and not having been more careful with her. In all of our years of marriage, I had never raised a hand to Trude, and now it pained me deeply to see that I may have inadvertently hurt her.

I gave her some medication to ease her evident discomfort. I had to powder it since lately she had been having trouble swallowing any pills, no matter how small. She had not had this problem long, but now I had found that crushing and burying the drug in jam or pudding made things easier.

I made a homemade splint and then quickly drove her to St. Joseph Hospital, a few blocks from our house. I asked to have her right wrist x-rayed, and even though I didn't know anyone on the hospital's staff, the personnel were quite responsive. They and I helped Trude to the x-ray room. She was afraid to have anyone to touch the injured arm, but I seemed to frighten her less than the strangers, so I had to assist the technician. After it was finished, I helped her back to the waiting room, cradling her right arm as gently as possible. I hoped the pain medication I had given her was strong enough to keep her comfortable.

The x-rays showed what I had feared: Both bones of her right forearm were broken at the wrist. I knew from experience with these types of breaks that she wouldn't be able to use her right hand for at least six weeks. I asked for a temporary wrist support to keep the bones more secure until I could get her in to see a good orthopedist.

During the drive back to our house, I didn't say much and Trude's silence seemed somehow different and more unhappy than the quietness to which I was becoming accustomed. When we first married, she used to give me the "silent treatment" when she was upset, but now it was hard to gauge if her silence meant anger or if she simply couldn't find the words.

After we got home, I called Dr. Terry Light, the chief of the Orthopedic Department at Loyola Medical Center, my parent hospital. I had consulted with him in the past concerning some of my patients. I also told him about Trude's behavior that caused the fall and he was very sympathetic. He asked about the pain and I told him I had given her an adequate dosage of medication and it seemed to be working as much as I could tell, given her lack of responsiveness. After setting up an appointment, I went to where Trude was resting and asked if she felt any better. She nodded but said nothing.

At the clinic, Dr. Light examined her thoroughly and she was prepared for the procedure by a nurse who injected an anesthetic into the injured area so Trude might have little or no pain when the bones were set.

As she lay on a cart in the operating suite, waiting for the cast, her right hand and arm were suspended by a series of tapes that were attached to a metal frame above her. Somehow—I still don't know how—her arm fell and hit the cart. She winced terribly. The pain of having her broken arm slam down like that must have been quite intense to make it past the local and oral painkillers she had received. I ran to her side and called for help. Once again I found myself quite angry at how badly things were turning out.

When it was time to have the cast applied, I sat next to her, holding her left hand. I don't think the casting hurt too much, for which I was thankful.

Why the accident happened was never answered, but apparently one of the straps wasn't hooked on as snugly as it should have been, and the weight of her arm pulled the whole apparatus loose. Everyone involved apologized, but there wasn't anything to be done about it after the fact. The next day, Dr. Light did another x-ray to check the alignment in the cast, and he noticed a problem above the fracture. He told me the bones were out of line, which could cause trouble later. It was most likely caused by her arm falling. Repairing it now would mean a lengthy operation, but her general health wasn't the best, and these visits to the hospital seemed to have traumatized her enough already. I elected to hold off on the surgery. In the long run, it may have been better to have had the operation right then rather than let the problem remain. I was to second-guess my decision each time I saw Trude holding her arm in an unnatural way which she did from then on. If the dementia were not so unpredictable there would have been no question but to operate right then.

As I drove home from the hospital, I thought about what might lie ahead of us. Just 15 months earlier the Alzheimer's had been diagnosed, and now it was moving in a direction that could be quite harmful to Trude and myself. I replayed the incident over and over, wondering what I could have done differently or what I could do to prevent another occurrence of an attack that might lead to more injury to either of us.

I had been doing lots of reading about Alzheimer's disease and even though I knew such outbursts were part of the general picture, I still longed to find a reason for the attacks. Of course there is no rational cause—the disease had made her behave this way. If she were living in the 19th century, she would have been called crazy and locked away indefinitely.

I vaguely remembered from years earlier a patient I had treated who had become violent when he descended through this stage of Alzheimer's. I knew that not only can there be aggressiveness, but that part of this bizarre picture could also include being depressed, agitated, responding to imaginary events, being unable to sleep, and wandering. The last problem—wandering, especially at night—is quite common and I had already prepared for this unwanted adventure by purchasing a SAFE bracelet so that if Trude somehow had wandered away without my noticing it, the identification number on it would allow anyone who found her to know where she belonged. It made me terribly sad to think I had to tag her as though she were a wayward pet, but I had heard too many stories of Alzheimer's patients blundering into traffic and being killed.

The cast proved an annoyance to Trude in almost everything she did. She tried using her left hand and got by. I made a clumsy attempt at most of the kitchen jobs she still did by rote.

On occasion I would ask her, "How does the arm feel, Babe?" And she might look at me and say, "Okay," or nothing, and I wasn't even sure the "Okay" had any meaning. She seemed unhappy, but never said much any more, so it was very hard to tell. Did she think I was responsible for her injury? I guess I couldn't blame her if she did.

Things settled down to an uneasy quiet for a few days, but then, six days after her cast was applied, things took another ugly turn. I had set the table in the way she always had done and was preparing dinner as best I could. Strangely, as far gone as the rest of her mind was, until the broken wrist she had still been performing most of the kitchen chores and would brush me out of the way if I interfered. I did feel the need to watch her in case she set a towel on the stove or something.

This evening, she had been resting on the sofa in the family room, but she could hear me moving about in the kitchen. I had my back to the breakfast room and was working at the counter when I heard her behind me. I turned just in time to see her coming at me with a knife in her left hand. She had apparently taken one of the knives from the setting that I had just put in place on the dining table. As she raised her left arm, I stopped her move and took the knife away from her. It was hard for her to resist since she wasn't used to using her left hand and couldn't fend me off with her broken right hand. I then led her back to the couch, helped her lie down and went to the phone. She was crying as I called an ambulance. I had her taken to the Loyola Medical Center and their psychiatric unit as an emergency admission. I was able to speak to the doctor on call, and he admitted her immediately.

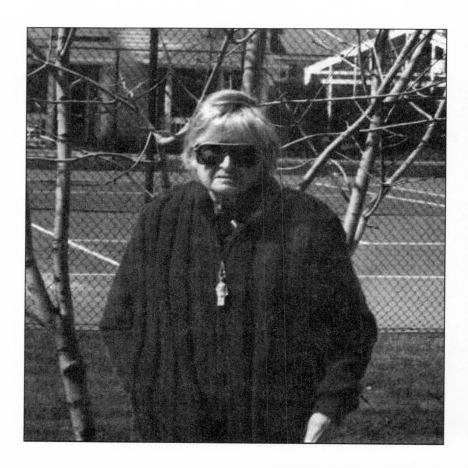

Trude near St. Patricks. (top)

Trude on a bench near the facility.

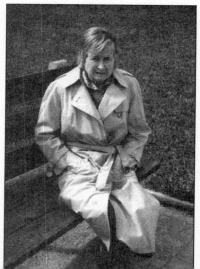

Looking for Help

I didn't know what else to do. Her behavior was becoming too erratic and dangerous. I was told I wouldn't be able to stay with her and that she would be medicated and kept for observation. I protested that it might be better if I stayed with her since she became uneasy around strangers and in unfamiliar surroundings, but the hospital staff insisted I leave. As I drove the 30 miles back to our house, I wondered if I had done the right thing for Trude or myself.

When I returned the next morning, she had been heavily medicated and was very quiet. I was pleased she'd been placed under the care of my friend, Dr. Bob De Vito, who was chairman of the Psychiatry Department.

Trude and I sat together in the lounge room and I tried to get her to talk, but she was sort of out of it, and she didn't really answer or react. By the next day it was apparent she had responded to her medicines and might be ready to go home in a couple of days. Before her discharge, Trude, Dr. De Vito and I sat in a conference room for at least an hour while he carefully reviewed her medical history. She sat impassively, silent during the whole discussion, and I again wondered if it was the drugs or her worsening condition that made her so quiet. Bob was pretty certain her diagnosis was Dementia Alzheimer Type and he assured me that my admitting her to the ward was necessary and was not uncommon with Alzheimer's dementia. This was the first time Trude needed any form of psychiatric care and, I hoped, the last.

While in the hospital, she was also seen by the orthopedic resident, who was called to change the cast. He applied a much more restrictive one, and I could see it was painfully interfering with her hand movements and causing her hand to tingle, so I later asked to have part of the cast cut away. But her hand still bothered her, mainly, I guess, due to the misalignment of the bones. Given her current state, an operation still was not possible.

Her mental condition had improved enough that she was to be discharged after the third day. Although she was a little groggy from the medication, I believed I could take care of her at home. The hospital's social service director warned me about what might be in store and that this might not be the best idea, since I didn't have the experience or training in caring for someone with dementia. He recommended a long-term-care nursing home, only a short drive from Joliet. After meeting with the admissions director there and taking a tour, I had Trude admitted to the specialized-care unit.

I talked to Trude about the move to another type of hospital where she could be helped and cared for and the break in her right wrist could heal faster. I told her I would be there to see her every day and she appeared to accept the change, but she was so passive and her vocabulary and emotions so limited, it was hard to tell.

The facility, St. Patrick's, was operated by a religious group and was located in Naperville, 20 minutes away from Joliet. I hadn't heard of it before, but it had been there a good number of years. The main building had a number of floors and was set on a large plot of land. Despite a lack of freeways going that direction, the drive on the back-country roads from Joliet to Naperville wasn't bad.

Once again I felt lost without Trude, and this time I feared more than last time that the separation might turn out to be permanent.

I visited her early in the afternoon each day, after she had tried to eat lunch with her left hand. The cast on the right arm impaired her every move since she didn't know how to cope with its uselessness. Trying to learn to do things with the wrong hand would be hard enough for any elderly person, but since Trude's mind wasn't fully functional, it compounded the difficulties.

I tried to spend as much time as possible with Trude, usually from noon until dinnertime. One day when I arrived on the floor I found a man sleeping in Trude's bed and her sitting in a chair next to her bed looking confused. Another time I found her closet empty. I went room to room and retrieved her things from various other closets. How her clothes came to be so scattered, I don't know. Her behavior was so erratic she may have moved them herself, or more likely, one of the other residents decided to do a little redecorating. During most of her time at St. Patrick's, she just lay in bed staring at the ceiling. It was very sad to watch this once-vibrant woman slipping further and further away.

As days went by, I noticed that often when I arrived on her floor, there were many residents milling about, coming and going from two other wards adjacent to Trude's. I guess I hadn't been looking too closely at the general surroundings when I checked things out, but calm and quiet seemed rare.

The staff would lead some of the residents in simple tasks such as passing a ball around a circle. Many other residents were just staring blankly at television sets. I doubt they would have reacted at all had I changed channels or simply shut off the sets. In even just the past few years, things have improved dramatically at this and other Alzheimer's care facilities, although they still have a long way to go, but back then not much was done for people who were given up as beyond hope and help.

Trude never tried any of the activities because of the cast, which was such a hindrance. Usually she would leave the lounge area and go back to her room and her bed. She waited for me to arrive to take her on our daily walk to the surrounding neighborhood, if the February weather permitted. There was no way to tell how long she would remain at St. Patrick's, but she would be there for at least six weeks, until she got the cast off. Since I was not even a competent cook, I assumed the nurses and the rest of the staff would be better able to assist her than I could.

One afternoon, as we got ready to go for our walk, I took her to the bathroom as I always did. She had to have some help, but this day I had trouble getting her slacks down, and when I finally did, I found she was wearing a diaper. My surprise turned to anger when the smell hit my nose, and I found that it was not only full, but from the looks of things had not been emptied in quite a while. Trude had been lying in bed before I came, suffering the annoyance of this unsanitary condition—never mind the embarrassment. I got her cleaned up and helped her back to bed.

I found the charge nurse on duty, and he didn't know who put the diaper on or who had ordered it. He assumed a nurse's aide on the morning shift had done so and failed to notify his staff at the change of shifts. I told him that it wasn't to happen again without a good reason and to notify me when I was on the unit. I was appalled at the insult to Trude's dignity and worried about the medical consequences of such a practice.

I suppose I overreacted, but I learned, to my disappointment, that not all long-term nursing-care facilities have specially trained personnel to care for people suspected of having Alzheimer's disease, and was surprised to see that many institutions like St. Patrick's mixed all stages of the illness in one unit. I still had much to learn about this disease, including what limited treatment options were available and what lay ahead for Trude.

The weeks turned into months, and her awareness continued to deteriorate. I wondered if her seemingly accelerated deterioration was due to the environment or the drugs, but never having had this much experience with anyone with this condition, I had no yardstick by which to gauge it.

With some help from the nurse, Trude had learned to eat with her left hand, but other than meals she spent most of her time in bed or in a chair in her room. Every day, we went for a walk in the neighborhood or for a ride in the car if the winter allowed us to do so, but sometimes even that was not possible, so all we could do was walk the corridors. Some of these walks were disturbing, since I could see the various sad stages to which a person could descend, and I had a hard time picturing Trude reduced to such a state.

We learned together what it meant for her to be living in a group of people who were losing their mental faculties, although Trude was unaware of most of what she was experiencing, which may have made it easier for her to cope with some of the humiliations. More than once, Trude's bed was occupied by a male resident, and I would come in to find her sitting in the chair next to her bed, not knowing what to do, waiting for him to leave. There were more instances when items of her clothing ended up in another woman's closet across the hall. The residents were often just scattered in the lounge—one was draped across an arm of a chair, another was asleep with his head drooped in a very uncomfortable position and another was pounding his fist on a lady's head as she sat in her wheelchair doing nothing, not even reacting to the assault.

With further checkups, it was apparent that Trude's arm wasn't going to heal properly, and this would hamper her in so many normal activities. That, plus the Alzheimer's dementia, meant she was going to be more and more dependent.

I wrote to Dr. Bob De Vito and tried to get a better understanding of what the future held for Trude. I explained to him that I was at a loss as to what to do now and in the months ahead.

He wrote back:

I think you are correct in your assessment of the deterioration of certain bodily functions. My reading on this is that Alzheimer's disease and related dementias are associated with a cascading loss of brain functions affecting a wide spectrum of psychological and behavioral activities. One might, or could see, a gradual yet progressive decline in logical thinking, judgment, problem solving, and real decision-making. Also, there is a degree of loss of sensation where body functions are involved. And as the disease goes on, loss of recognition of one's self and familiar objects which were easily identifiable in the past. An Alzheimer-affected person may manifest progression with

their brain damage affecting a broad array of behavioral reactions, anywhere
from being a recluse to aggressive assaulting behavior episodes.

It was a depressing prognosis, to say the least. Each night when I would arrive back at the house in Joliet, I would go to our favorite spot in the family room, sit in my lounge chair, close my eyes and remember. So many things went through my mind. I even called out to her one evening, "This is what it used to be like."

In one of his frequent phone calls, our son, Rick, suggested I move his mother back to California and into a center that was devoted exclusively to the care of those suspected of having Alzheimer's dementia. Ms. Ferri Kidane was the chief operating officer at the John Douglas French Center in Los Alamitos, and she had been Rick's patient. She said she could arrange for the admission. I still had the condominium where I could stay, and, although it would mean a good deal of driving, I could see no alternative.

The French Center was founded by Dorothy Kirsten French, an opera singer whose husband, neurosurgeon John Douglas French, had died of Alzheimer's. She built the center in hopes of having a decent place to care for her husband; the doors opened in February, 1988, and Dr. French died in 1989. As the first Alheimer's care center in the world, it has been widely emulated. Towards the end, Dr. French could barely move and couldn't speak, but his wife sang to him and played music for him in hopes that something could penetrate his stupor.

At the French Center, they don't use any official stages to rank residents, but do try to group like-functioning people together. There are six suites housing the different groups, and each suite is named for roles Mrs. French had performed. Trude was assigned to the Violetta suite, along with 20 other women and men.

I got us first-class tickets to cut down on Trude's anxiety about being surrounded by strangers, and we flew to California the first week in May.

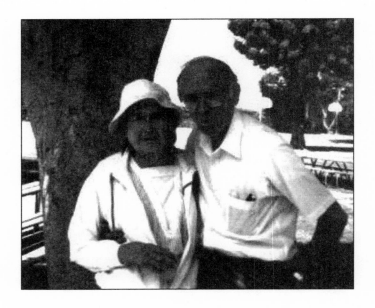

Trude and I in Southern
California. (top)

Our friends Russ and Jean
Stevens.

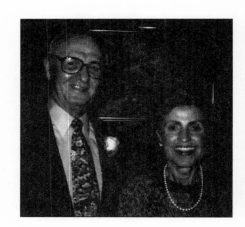

Back to Southern California

Trude had a small private room, similar to one you'd find in a hospital. Outside each room there was a memory box that held the resident's photo and a few small personal items to remind the resident and the staff who this person was. Trude was under fairly constant care and observation by either the nursing supervisor or the assistants. She usually ate with the other residents in the suite, except as time went on she would stay in her room and needed help with eating.

Some of the higher-functioning residents were on drugs, but most weren't, because past a certain point no available drug helps. And for many the drugs just seemed to bring them back to a level where they were aware of what they were losing. We discussed what medications might be beneficial for Trude, but other than the one that controlled her violent tendencies, I had vetoed any of the others. Some were like using a garden hose on a rapidly advancing forest fire, and I was afraid of others that might have too many side effects. With Trude's limited ability to communicate, she couldn't tell us if something was wrong. We were fortunate that both Rick and I were physicians, and although neither of us specialized in psychiatry or neurology, we were better able to follow the increasingly complex situation than I am sure some lay people would have been.

John Bayley noted that when he tried a new drug for his wife that was supposed to slow the advance of Alzheimer's, "the friendly fog suddenly dispersed, revealing a precipice before her feet." He quickly discontinued the medicine.

The only medication we tried with Trude was the female hormone estrogen as part of a study since some research had suggested it might help. It didn't. Another drug we tried was Vitamin E, which some say can slow the disease.

The French Center has room for about 130 residents and is handsomely furnished, with nice amenities, including a library and Internet access for the higher-functioning residents. Considering the sad state of the residents, most seemed rather happy. As Ms. Kidane said, many have the thrill of experiencing everything with childlike wonder, for, in a sense, they are seeing a flower or bird or hearing a joke or seeing a movie for the first time, since they have no prior memory of it.

The facility has an aviary, a garden and some rooms available for private parties. Trude made a good deal of use of the putting green. Strange that with all the other things she had lost, Trude could still putt. They use lots of aromatherapy, particularly in the suite where people tend to be violent. Various scents seem to calm them. The lights are dimmed at mealtime to try to calm the violent residents, and they adjust the lights in the evening to try to counteract "sundowning." The staff is taught how to restrain residents without hurting them. They have learned that most of the violent spells are triggered by something like a loud noise, bright light or the patient being reminded of someone else, in which case they have found it might be necessary to keep a caregiver away from a certain resident. They have tried to make the facility as safe and peaceful as possible, but given the unpredictability of behavior, there are still episodes.

I would visit her every day and take her out for a walk. The Southern California weather was much less limiting than what we faced in Illinois. When I would arrive, she was already dressed and I would say, "Let's go out dear." Often we would go to the ocean, since Seal Beach was only a five-minute drive, or we'd walk down Katella Avenue, the heavily trafficked main street on which the French Center was located. Trude would hold my left arm tightly against her, which seemed to help make her feel secure. Sometimes we walked to a quiet schoolyard around the corner or to the gazebo in a ministry site that was a short walk from the school. At the schoolyard we would sit and I would tell her what I had been doing, although I was never sure how little she was comprehending. Sometimes she would nod as though she were following me, but most of the time she stared off into space. Children running by would catch our attention for a moment as they headed home, and I would tell Trude how much I missed her, as if she didn't know already or perhaps had forgotten how much I loved her. One day, a woman came by and said hello. She saw the camera hanging from my neck and presumed we were tourists, and she offered to take our photo. She took a couple photos and went on her way.

Trude seemed to like the walks along the pier in Seal Beach and to dig her toes into the sand. She liked to feel the waves lap around her feet and ankles and would look out to sea. I wondered if she was seeing the beautiful beach scene before her eyes today or was lost in the memory of some past time. On some of these strolls, I would bring along a beach pad, and she enjoyed lying down and resting there with the peaceful drone of the ocean waves in the background. I took a photograph of her sleeping there one day. This photo, along with the ones that woman took at the schoolyard, are about the last ones I have before the disease really took its toll on Trude's features.

From May through September of 1995, I took the daily drive from the condominium in Rancho Bernardo, in San Diego County, to Los Alamitos, 87 miles away, close to where Orange County meets Los Angeles County, just east of Long Beach.

I wrote a letter to Russ and Jean Stevens about one of my long commutes:

> Friends:
>
> I think I may be overdoing the traveling a bit. I fell asleep at the wheel on the way home as I was driving down Interstate 5 just beyond San Onofre Beach area, but fortunately the road ahead was wide and I caught myself in time. I then headed for the closest exit and sat in a parking lot overlooking the Pacific until I thought I was awake. I still had to drive to Oceanside and

then across 78 to 15 and to the condo. Obviously, I made it without further
mishap.

Trude is unchanged. I feel her overall outlook is dimmer each day since I
don't think she can be taken off the drugs to slow her down and that just
makes her less responsive. She's between a rock and a hard place.

Whether I will continue to make the trip daily is a large question I cannot answer yet. She doesn't really know me, I don't believe, and if she does
have any recognition of me, it's not very real. It makes me so angry, I would
tear the facility down if I were able.

Also, would you believe one of her brown loafer shoes is missing. And I
am paying $5,250 a month for expert care. Give me a break. I told the nurs-
ing supervisor how I felt and I said I've already had this type of experience
at the last place. Is this a universal problem?

My main project now is the videotape film biography on Trude that I am
arranging for a production company down the road in Miramar. I'm compil-
ing about 300–400 pictures and music from those old days—songs we both
liked and some from today. I particularly like "Perhaps Love" by John
Denver and of course "Memories on a Piano Solo."

Over the last month I have been re-reading our old letters and I am now
in 1943—February. I have come to a conclusion and that is . . . I never
should have married her. A prime reason was her superior intelligence which
I thwarted in a way by courting her and then convincing her to become Mrs.
Z. Also, I keep realizing this girl was a WOMAN and I was an immature
child. The difference in our ages and her experience in the business world for
3–4 years before we wed; her good looks and figure and her innate ability to
do things well, and the attention she drew from other men never showed up
as it has at this time in the letters. If I was older when we did carry on in
the '40s I would never have tolerated her shenanigans. It seemed she just had
to be doing something with someone be it male or female, and usually the
former during the week to stem the "loneliness" from me since I was only
able to date her on the weekends. I think in our letters if she made that point
once about seeing me on Saturday and partly on Sunday (I had to go back to
Chicago and to school that nite) and why not more often than that she said it

50x. And of course, what the hell does a 20 year old punk whose infatuated with this marvelous young lady do...he lets it go. She wore my ring and wore my frat pin and still that didn't mean hoodly-do. She still went out. The next letter would describe her antics and then, all of these gushy words of love and forever yours. Boy, how naïve can a guy be. And it really annoys me now even though she settled down somewhat when she worked in Chicago that year before we tied the knot. I saw her very often then which may have allayed that "loneliness" somewhat.

It might have been better for her also if she had joined the WAVES as she threatened to do to see the world and be patriotic. Maybe she could have married a big wheel officer and been an Admiral's wife. I think that is why she went to work at the USO...the boys.

As you can tell I ain't in a very good mood today.

But I still love her. How can I not after all this time. It just seems that what I must have thought about this affair was like the movies we went to. Boy sees girl; boy meets girl; boy marries girl. Not here Charley. She was an entirely different woman. I wish she would have been able to go on to a higher education since I am convinced she would have been somebody and accomplished it well. Maybe if she had used all brain cells in learning more and more there would have been no room for Alzheimer's to destroy her— and me.

Z

I was having the video done for Trude's 75th birthday, but knew she wouldn't be well enough by then to have any idea what was happening, so started it a bit early. I guess part of me thought that if I could find a way to connect to her past that maybe one or both of us would have something to hang on to as the present got worse.

I thought it would be great to ask for reflections from her old class-mates and co-workers extending back to the 1940s. I knew only a handful of the women to whom I addressed my request, but most responded. The video was to tell the story of her life, from early childhood until the onset of her illness.

I was gratified by the many kind responses I received:

She was one of the prettiest and nicest persons I've ever known.
Adrianna Reato Vidmar.

I remember well the Herald News time-change photo. Trude did no brag-
ging. She somewhat shyly told us of the subsequent invitation from you. We
were delighted and wondered what it might lead to. What a love story.
Jeanette Nystrom Westberg

She was such a sweetheart. She was intelligent without being arrogant.
She was such a pretty girl but didn't flaunt it. She had a wonderful sense of
humor and was a good friend during our teen years.
Helen Gerl Kachel

I used to see Trude and admired her. I was just a skinny blonde that no
one noticed, and she was beautiful.
Margaret Keller Ashbaugh

I've known her from grade school and high school. She was a very smart
girl in grammar school. She had her hands in different things. She was in a
lot of plays in school.
Mary Pariza Kargus

The only thing I can contribute about Trude is that I remember her as a
very nice, beautiful and happy young Lady and I capitalize the word Lady
as she was every bit that.
Elizabeth Przybylski Latek

I moved to Joliet in 1938, six weeks after school had started. It was the
senior year and I had to carry about eight subjects to graduate due to differ-
ent requirements. I remember Trudy as being one of the few people who
spoke to me in a friendly way. Joliet is a very clicky town.
Evon Jones Keck

When I read these compliments, they didn't amaze me since I knew all of those things about her—but that each of these women could recall those special features about Trude 55 years later did. I found myself looking back with nostalgia, because to look forward more than one day at a time was too painful. The hope that the void might lessen was just wishful thinking.

As my letter to Russ and Jean reflected, I was also not entirely happy with the French Center, but I guess I just wanted everything to be perfect for Trude. But that might have been a bit unrealistic, since dealing with so many people with such an unpredictable illness means things can't stay perfect long.

Each day, with my visit to Trude, I would notice the ways the residents were carrying on: one sleeping in a chair, another jabbering in a nonsensical way, another pacing the halls without an obvious goal in sight, another sitting on a sofa holding the hand of one of the other residents with an occasional movement to try a kiss. Even Trude used to pace with no definite purpose, but with such a forceful step that it seemed as if she were bound for an urgent destination only she could see.

As at St. Patrick's, often Trude and other people would be found in the wrong beds. In spite of having a photo of the resident posted next to his or her door, the residents were often incapable of recognizing their own room. They did have various activities, including dances, but Trude rarely participated in these. In fact, she and I only danced at one dance for about two minutes and then she never wanted to again, and never did. This particularly depressed me, remembering how she loved to dance and what a good dancer she was. How sad that she could be robbed of the memory of even that simple pleasure.

About a month after she arrived, I was getting ready for our afternoon trip to the beach and she was in her room, lying in bed. As I bent over her to change her socks, out of the corner of my eye I caught a person moving toward me from the open doorway of her room, just behind me. It was one of the male residents, who came at me and kicked my right thigh. I jumped away and started after him as he hurried out of the room and down the corridor.

I went to the nursing station to tell of the attack, and while I was telling the nurse what happened, he came at me again. One of the male nursing assistants intervened and took the resident to his room. I demanded to know what was going on. The nurse said, "We have this happen occasionally, but he'll settle down."

I angrily told them to get him off the floor and away from Trude. He was taken to another suite that night.

I had seen this same man, who was of average build and appeared to be over 65 years of age, trying to be overly sociable with some of the women. He always had a blank, hard look about him. While sitting on a lounge sofa, he would often edge close to a woman and place his arm around her neck.

During the one dance we attended, this same man was moving around as though he was interested in something besides the music. After he attacked me, I wondered if he was jealous of my being so close to Trude. Although I didn't need to be reminded, when I discussed the incident with Ms. Kidane, she said that Alzheimer's doesn't necessarily shut down the part of the brain that controls sexual desire and performance, and that men seem to maintain their libido longer than women, as is the case with older people who don't have the disease. Of course, since he may be incapable of recognizing his own spouse, problems can arise.

Before Trude's illness, our intimacy was always wonderful, and now I found it frustrating to be so close to her as I held her to lift her into or out of bed and not be able to do more than kiss her or stroke her cheek. She never initiated anything beyond that, and since she was no longer able to consent, I never went any further.

On occasion, I'd ask her, "Baby Dear, can you say, 'I love you?'" and she'd repeat the words to me in a slightly garbled way, with a thickened smothering. And even though it wasn't that clear, when she did try to respond, I felt a surge of love for her I cannot describe. At the same time I felt a painful torment when I heard those words and wonder how much worse it must have been for her if she was at all aware of what was happening.

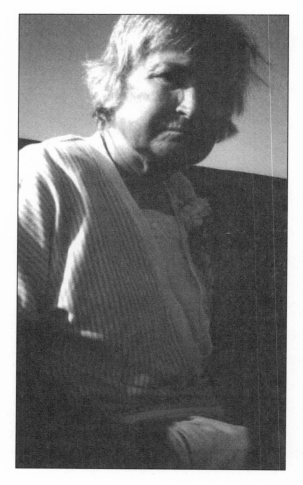

Trude on our anniversary in Southern California. (top)

Trude and her sister Ag at the condo in Rancho Bernardo.

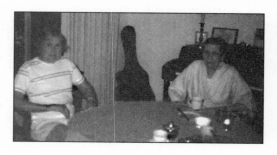

Back to Illinois

I wrote another letter to the Stevenses, again pouring out my troubles to my dear old friends:

Today is the 7th

Greetings from foggy San Diego:

Just started to type this out when the mail arrived with your letter.

Still haven't played golf but it seems you do nothing but, old boy. The joints will suffer with too much activity. And how about your favorite back ache. Rub him in every night, Jean, with my favorite, Ben Gay. It works.

The condo remains in disorder. The rugs need cleaning and a kitchen cabinet shelf tipped after I installed it to hold a few pieces of glassware... I still don't know why it tipped. Maybe we had an earthquake while I was gone??? Broke a teapot.

As I have indicated my vision isn't very good and if all goes according to schedule, the Shiley Eye Clinic eye surgeon should have completed the removal of the cataract from the right one by the time you receive this letter. Friday was to be the day of the surgery.

Hope this outfit is competent. Am concerned when I'll be able to drive since there is a varied opinion from this and that one.

Traveling here, there, and everywhere. Would you believe I have put on 7000 miles since I arrived. But everything seems at a distance.

Trude's film biography is slowly coming about and I hope it will be nice for Rick and Judy and the grandkids. It's not easy to recapitulate on memories and a few facts but I'll complete it eventually.

I may be moving her down to El Cajon soon. Her care wherever she is remains the same. Visited a home there and it is 30 miles away. As I said nothing is close. Decisions, decisions.

I stay pretty well inactive and phone calls are a main source of keeping in touch. And as I've said, I'm supposed to get on with living but that's easier said than done. Maybe I should go down to the naval base and see if I can steal a cruiser and drive up the coast. Hell, the fellow who stole the tank ended up on the 163 freeway—I've been on it frequently on the way to San Diego itself. If I can ever accept the disease Trude has been struck with then maybe I'll settle down. Try to understand what it means to have her so and totally unable to converse and what it means to have her in a hospital setting where there is absolutely nothing to look forward to each day.

Memorial Day is tomorrow and I may put the flag up, if I have the energy and verve to do so.

Adieu (as Trude would say) until we write or speak again. If I do fall asleep at the wheel and I hit the jackpot, tell them I was a nice kid in 1942 and grew up slower than the others.

Clearly my own mental and physical state was deteriorating. In the letter I made reference to the big news that a man had stolen a tank and had gone on a mad joyride through the streets and down the freeways of San Diego before being shot by the police. I had so little to do other than the long and taxing drives to Los Alamitos which gave me much too much time to think about what a sad direction our lives were heading. I would look forward to my visits with Trude and then be freshly disappointed each time I would see her in her present state.

A little later, I typed another note of woe to Russ and Jean:

August 7, 1995

Russ and Jean:

It is Sunday and I am readying myself to go north again. Am also driving a rental car—courtesy of the Olds agency.

A few cursory observations:

The drivers in California must have no fear of anything including the highway patrol. Me neither. If I get stopped I'll fight the charge to the

Supreme Court. Of course, yesterday on the Pacific Coast Highway, a news-
man met his fate and the van looked like a train had hit it.

Along the stretch of Int. 5 just before the Oceanside city exit 78 is
reached there is a field of produce growing. I wish I could stop and see what
it is. The entire plot of land—and I measured it with my odometer, is 13
blocks long and I imagine 6 blocks deep going toward the ocean, is staked.
I'll bet there are at least thousands of 3 feet poles in line as far as the eye can
see with a wooden brace to the ground in support. There's a wee amount of
green growth coming up now and the produce may be beans. But it's amaz-
ing. What patience to put those poles in the ground one by one.

Time moves on inexorably and Trude has been at the center now three
months. Whether I'll continue her care there is uncertain. She hurt herself
again and fortunately didn't break anything. She fell against the end table
next to her bed as she tried to get into the bed after having been showered.
Her feet were wet and she was trying to get away from the caregiver with
the fall as a result. I got there a short time later and the nurse informed me
of what had happened. Every time the phone rings now I pick it up with
much trepidation. Also, the psychiatrist increased her agitation drug to 3x a
day so now I can expect her to be like a zombie again.

We go out each day if she wants to. Didn't go anywhere after the fall,
and I don't know what to expect in general since she can't tell me. Now she
just wants to walk & walk. Went to the beach but I can't get her to sit any
more than 30 seconds to enjoy the sea air and the people and the ocean.

My days are like yours but maybe you two kids get less bored than I do. I
did my shirts this AM; washed Trude's slacks and panties (will return
today): fought an onslaught of ants with RAID and I think I won, and try
to decide where to go and what to do.

Am almost finished with the film project material. Going down to the
producer this week and try to get everything in order. Even though she won't
know what it is all about, maybe the music will stir her memories.

Less than a week after the fall that I had described to Russ and Jean, I
again got a call, this time because of a deep cut over Trude's right elbow.
No one knew how it happened, but a doctor saw her and prescribed

antibiotics. I got reports from the center that Trude at times was combative and difficult. It hurt so much to have my sweet Trude described that way, and to think that her own unruly behavior might be the cause of some of her injuries was really disturbing.

With my drive to visit every day, seven days a week, for months, I started to falter physically. Not knowing what else to do, I checked Trude out of the center. I explained my reason to Ms. Kidane, who tried to warn me of just how hard it would be for me to care for Trude on my own. Perhaps it was the long drives or just my naïveté that made me think this was a good move.

As stupid as it now seems for a medical person to be thinking this, I guess back then I still believed that Trude's was a temporary problem that would somehow disappear, like a cold or a headache, if given the time.

The plan was that Trude and I would live in the condominium in Rancho Bernardo, where I would again try to take care of her. As I thought about it, and to make the move more secure, I again phoned her eldest sister, Agatha, now 76 years old, and asked her to fly to California and help out.

Now that I was with Trude 24 hours a day, I became even more painfully aware of how impaired her reasoning was and just how difficult it was to communicate with her.

Sometimes crying or grimacing was her way of saying something was wrong and she needed help, and at other times there was no discernable cause. It was like dealing with an infant—guessing at the reasons for the crying, and once you had solved the obvious ones—the need for the bathroom or food—I felt like a young parent stymied when the reason for the crying was not apparent.

By now she had stopped talking completely, and I missed the sound of her voice.

Over the first four weeks, even with Ag's help, it was quite difficult. I could see the situation was taking a toll on Ag, so I hired nurse's aide to assist me. Finding a good one wasn't easy. Why I thought it might be easier to take care of Trude than to drive to see her, I don't know, other than my exhaustion may have reduced my own decision-making abilities. I began to feel I would need to look for more consistent and expert care again, but the experiences at St. Patrick's, the Remington Club, and even the French Center, had me concerned about trying again. She got so frightened without me that I hesitated to put her in another institution.

In the last few years, care facilities have improved dramatically, and the amount of information available to caregivers has increased phenomenally. But in 1995, I often felt like I was breaking new ground, and had nowhere to turn for advice.

While we lived at the condominium, I made notes frequently to see if I could find a way to set up a better care plan, and the notes say almost as much about my mental state as they do about Trude's.

Friday the 6th Oct. '95. Slept well last night. Awoke at 7 a.m. Ate breakfast. Nurse arrived—not very helpful since I did everything for Trude. Dulcolax suppository, a bowel stimulant, used with results in bed—unfortunately. I wonder whether there is a brain reaction to the chemical makeup of the Dulcolax since Trude was out of sorts most of the day. Went to the store late in the afternoon and she tolerated it well. The same day, a most frightening experience occurred just as we finished the meal. For no reason that was plain to me, she grabbed the napkin on the table and before I could grasp what she was trying to do, she started to put it in her mouth. I had to forcibly remove the bitten piece of paper, fearful she could have choked on it. This made her more upset. Went to bed at 10 pm and she slept all night awakening at 7 am.

Up and down with combative behavior.

The nurse is too pushy and cooks gourmet foods; sits on the patio porch and smokes cigarettes, also coughs a lot. Talks too loud.

Trude's eyes are wild and it may mean another aggressive attack on me or the nurse.

Medication makes no difference.

Her night was marred by many trips to the bathroom and occasional urine deposits in the bowl. Fell in bathroom injuring right forearm. But I don't know how she fell or why. I looked her over carefully and no obvious signs of anything bad. Will watch closely.

Dinner eaten but up and down haphazardly. Went to bed and to bathroom 10x. Awake at 3 am. Seemed combative and hard to control.

Brushes teeth fairly well. I had to use Dulcolax suppository today as usual but then had a clean-up.

The day was quiet. Three doses of Haldol were given rather than the usual two. She seemed to walk haltingly but we made it.

Ate breakfast but I needed to assist her.

Drove the nurse to the bus stop nearby and she is gone. Probably, one of the worst adventures in our stay at the condominium.

Sat and listened to music for an hour then she headed for the bedroom.

We went out to the store and the bank. Gone one-half hour.

There is a strange event occurring at intervals with Trude. She seems to get flushed and her skin is hot all over. Pulse rate is up to 96–100. And I checked her temperature by mouth, rectally, and the armpit, which is always a degree lower than by mouth. The reading today was .4 degrees over normal. At the same time she fixes her gaze into space, blinking her eyes almost never. Part of this sudden change is accompanied with a tone of belligerence. Then, it disappears 1–2 hours later.

I don't feel her home care is going to be effective, and more unlikely in any facility. Her disease is too far gone centrally.

Into bed at 9:30 pm. Snoring away. A different scenario entirely.

Went out shopping at Nordstrom's to buy her new clothes—to the drug store for a commode seat—to the grocery store where she wheeled the cart. And she was fine. Ate dinner and rested. Into bed at 9:30 pm.

I'm definitely concerned about her urine difficulty. I don't know whether it's drug related or disease related.

Bad, bad day all around.

Went out for walk—10 minutes or so. She struggles to walk and her inability to do so becomes more obvious each day. Drug? Disease? Hard to tell what.

With the increasing difficulties, my hope that we could continue to live here was evaporating. If a decent nursing assistant could be found, the task might be manageable, but without one, it looked impossible. It was apparent that Trude's care was becoming more and more unpredictable and there was only an occasional letup. The drug, Risperdal, prescribed by a psychiatrist she saw while we were at the condominium, was to quiet her down in a different way than the Haloperidol, or "Haldol," that Dr. DeVito had prescribed to keep her quiet and stop any agressiveness. The downside of the Haldol was that it quieted her to an almost zombie-like state. The choice remained whether to have her sort of spaced-out most of the time or have her mood swings which could become violent. It wasn't too much longer before both medications were stopped.

In November I decided to go back to Joliet. I was having my own health problems: I had a minor operation and had to see a heart specialist and thought it might be better to be back home again where I knew the hospitals and doctors to care for both of us. I supposed my running back and forth to California on some subconscious level was a feeble attempt at running away from our problems—for a while I felt that if I could find the right place Trude would be better there.

It was clear now. There was no right place, and Trude would never be better.

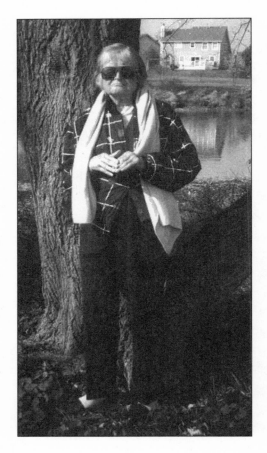

Trude on one of our walks in Joliet. (top)

Trude after her injury.

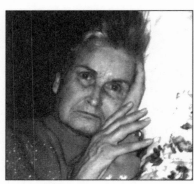

Sad Homecoming

When we got back, we again stayed at the home of Trude's sister Ann and her husband Jack Phalen, in Plainfield, about six miles from our last address in Joliet. We planned to stay with them until our new home was finished.

I had hired an engineering firm to design a custom home to accommodate Trude's special needs. There would be ramps instead of stairs into the house, and at the rear there would be a large outdoor deck easily accessible from several rooms. We planned rounded corners where two walls came together so there would be no sharp edges to pose a danger. Electrical outlets would be capped, and the stove would have a protective cover. The idea fell through when I realized I didn't have the five months or more it would take to complete the work.

Trude's care was becoming more difficult and I realized I couldn't go on imposing on Jack and Ann much longer, and upsetting their lives. Rather than try to go on with her caregiving myself, since my own health was shaky—I was having chest pains and still having eye trouble—I thought it would be better to have her admitted to another health-care center. I chose one called the Wealshire, which had just opened about 50 miles from Plainfield. This was supposed to be a better, more innovative sort of nursing facility with the latest in amenities for elder care.

The 100-mile round trip was hard on me, since my vision and my chest pains were getting worse, but it was still not as bad as the drive to the French Center had been. I would always enjoy being with

Trude, and we'd take walks in and around the garden areas when we were able or take a ride to a nearby park, weather permitting. I usually undertook the slow task of feeding her lunch and dinner while the record player spun out the old standards for everyone in the dining room.

The situation at the Wealshire didn't get off to a good start; within 10 days of her admission, things started to go wrong. After I thought I had Trude properly situated, I flew back to California to arrange to have the condo cleaned and see about renting it out. I called as soon as I got there on Friday to make sure everything was fine, and it was. When I called two days later, I was told that Trude had fallen and had a bruise on the right side of her head and two black eyes. They didn't know how the fall had occurred, and no one had bothered to notify me, although Judy and the attending physician had been called. When the nurse described Trude's current condition, I jumped on the first plane back.

I went straight to the Wealshire and took Trude to the nearest hospital for a thorough exam and an x-ray of her skull, something that the staff apparently never thought to do. A skull fracture was confirmed by a neurosurgeon, but it was rather difficult to assess the damage since her lack of response to many of the tests that were routinely used to determine the extent of a concussion could have been due to the Alzheimer's.

Since Trude had other falls at other places, I guess I didn't blame the Wealshire as much as I should have and was too forgiving about their failure to have sought immediate medical attention for her. Or maybe it was my own exhaustion that let me return Trude to their care.

Only a few days later, I had just returned home from feeding Trude her dinner when I got a phone call from the staff saying Trude had fallen again. Again they didn't know how it had happened, but she had a cut to her face that was bleeding badly, and she had also bruised her nose very badly. I nearly killed myself rushing back there. When I got there, she was lying in bed with no one attending to her. I ordered an ambulance and had her taken to Loyola Hospital. She was kept there for three days and was to have problems with the tear sac under her left eye from then on.

I may be a slow learner, but clearly a return to the Wealshire was out of the question now. I had accepted that falls are part of the picture for an elderly person with dementia, but the staff's seeming ignorance of what to do for an injured person frightened me.

I was busy seeing to Trude's medical care and my own and didn't have time to look for a place, so Trude's sister, Ann, who understood what I wanted to accommodate Trude's special needs, looked at a few places and chose one suitable. The home she picked was all on one level, with only one step up into it from the outside, that could be easily ramped for a wheelchair. It had a large room that was the family, living and dining rooms all in one. I thought this was good, so I could keep an eye on Trude and she would still have space to roam. It was the model home for a new subdivision on the west side of Joliet. We moved in December 8, 1995.

Sooner than I had planned, I had to throw myself into the task of being Trude's primary caregiver. I had learned much in the past year and still had much to learn about caring for someone so incapacitated but came to believe I could do at least as good a job as the facilities that claimed to be skilled in these things. If nothing else, she would be my only concern. I could pay close attention to her, but I wasn't a trained nurse or nurse's aide and had found I had much to learn about caring for someone's every need. Nurses often complain that the doctor leaves the room before the dirty work starts, and now I was learning what it meant to perform every aspect of someone's care. I knew this time I had to do the job right no matter what, because resorting to another care facility seemed the quickest route to another serious injury for Trude. I immediately started looking for a nurse's aide and a housekeeper to assist me in the big job I had undertaken. In the meantime, I had to try to learn to see to meals and do the household chores myself, which was not an easy task for one as underskilled in such arts. I gained a new appreciation for the ease with which Trude had performed myriad tasks over the years.

I also tried to prepare the house for Christmas. After the children had grown and flown we had scaled back on our decorating, but while Trude was well she still liked a tree and lights and the manger that I'd had since I was a child. I had been given this beautiful stable and figures that had been handmade by a man who worked for my father. Its craftsmanship always caught the attention of anyone who visited our home during the holidays, and I hoped that such touches would stir some glimmer of recognition in Trude. As December wore on, I began to doubt that Trude had the slightest idea what season it was and wondered if I had wasted a lot of effort on lights that she was too ill and I too depressed to appreciate. My heart wasn't really in it anymore as I dug out a small ceramic Christmas tree which had been given to me years earlier by a grateful patient. In years past, Trude had admired the way that so much cheer could emanate from this foot-high tree and the brightness that shone from its tiny multi-colored lights. Now its effect was lost on her.

My Christmas letter in 1996 recapped some of the events of the intervening 12 months:

> Our house was a busy place with housekeepers coming and going. So hard to find a good one. And finding a good nurse-assistants has also been taxing. I had a 75th birthday party for Trude, although she was not well enough to appreciate the gathering of family and friends. I showed the film of her life "A Girl Name Trude." We also had a 52nd anniversary party which offered a chance to see a lot of the same friends who attended our 50th, but now Trude was completely oblivious to their presence.
>
> Ron was working on his train set-up with David's help as usual.
>
> Rick retired and his wife continues writing, mainly on subjects about Native Americans.

Trying to keep good help was difficult and frustrating. I had one show up drunk, and another I caught drinking on the job. Some seemed to think their job description consisted primarily of sitting outside smoking cigarettes.

I typed up a list of Trude's activities to try to give them some idea of what to expect:

Trude is usually ready to rise at 7 a.m. She will lie in her bed until assisted from it. She has a tendency to wind herself in her bedclothes. Upon getting out of bed, I hold her to be sure she has her balance. (It is not the greatest.)

To the bathroom to sit on the toilet is the next step.

She cannot brush her teeth on her own so I have her hold the brush and paste with me directing the movement of the brush. I then wash her, step by step. During this time I always have my arm behind her in case she steps backward which is a frequent problem.

Each day I select clothes that are color coordinated. (She was a very careful dresser no matter where she was going or what she was doing.)

Breakfast is normally no problem. Feeding her any food is time consuming. Only small amounts of anything are given since she has a tendency to chew a piece of anything 2–3x and then stop, holding the morsel in her left cheek area. Any liquid, again only in sips is helpful to let her swallow the food. While she is eating, she may hold her lips tight—this may be due to the fact that she is ready to burp 2 or 3x. Most all food is consumed. She weighs 148–150 pounds.

She will then lie on the couch since there is no other thing to do. May rest quietly staring into space. I usually put music on for her.

In mid-morning, we may go out for a walk (weather permitting) or to the store in the car.

Lunch is usually a docile event, but not always. She may be restless and moves her arms about, holding the feeder's arm. May also want to get up from the table. I resist her desire. Again, feeding is a long process.

The afternoon offers nothing in activity until 3 or 4 when a ride to the mall is made and a walk takes 30–40 minutes. Before or after, we may make a side trip in the car which she tolerates well—up to a couple of hours—no more.

When evening arrives, the behavior varies from cooperation to combativeness and restlessness. Up and down off the couch; turning and tossing; holding on to one's hand with a tight grip.

Feeding may be difficult, but can be done. Caution is suggested so there is no chance for aspiration.

Feeding takes at least 45 mins. After dinner, a short walk ensues—10–15 min only. And back to the couch. She may fall asleep or lie quietly. There are restless periods at times—wanting to get off the sofa and slip to the floor. She may just lie there or try to arise. This latter act is where her falls have occurred—fortunately, there have been no fractures or less serious damage sustained.

If she does fall asleep quite soundly, I never awaken her since if she is alarmed, showing fear and will not cooperate to retire to the bedroom. I wait and talk to her quietly trying to allay her anxiety.

I occasionally will get her pajamas on early to avoid a need later on. A diaper is used at bedtime. I rarely use it during the day unless a suppository (Dulcolax) has been used that morning. Dulcolax acts in 15–40 mins and also affects urination as well. I have learned the critical results with Dulcolax may not be the only action. Wait 60–75 mins before dressing her again.

On the day the suppository is used, the behavior is erratic. Her restlessness and agitation is in the p.m. It is variable. On & off the sofa—wanting to go to the front door and look out; occasionally pushing and pulling—(she has great strength). All of these manifestations may last one or more hours then stop. She sleeps most all night and hardly ever gets out of bed by herself. She snores a lot and has cycles of sleep apnea. (The not uncommon problem many people have of stopping breathing momentarily while sleeping. This wakes them and they fall right back to sleep.)

I believe her thermo-regulatory center is faulty because of the skin heat generated. With that comes an elevated pulse, restlessness, and tenseness of her jaw muscles. And her grasp is almost unbreakable.

Her wild-eyed, starry look is frequent and her cooperation is flawed at that time. Better to leave her alone.

Walking is usually not a problem but at times she veers rightward with her head directed to the right as well. If left on her own to move that way, she will fall—her propulsion is uncontrollable. In walking, her depth perception is bad—misses stepping over impediments easily. This effect of her exercise seems to occur only when outside—walk indoors.

The recurrent urinary tract infection is difficult to appreciate since she cannot voice distress and I'm sure there is some to a marked degree at times. If she cries with passage of urine, a specimen should be obtained.

She does not swallow a pill or capsule or anything else without chewing it first. So all Rx has to be powdered and mixed with a semi-liquid substance (cereal, ice cream).

Participation in activities is minimal.

My greatest concern is her falling. And her pushing someone else—not maliciously, but because she is going somewhere.

Two major concerns of mine are the sudden tendency to cry and appear to be in abdominal distress and 2) sudden onset of increased skin heat, increase in pulse and a tendency to hyperventilate. This latter event is an hour long and then disappears.

It was a complete and completely depressing picture of life for an Alzheimer's patient. The list of activities included walks almost daily and on these I would encounter many of the patients I or my brother Joe had treated in town. My family's lingering prominence had made me a bit of a local celebrity as well, so people recognized me and Trude on our outings. The tellers at the bank or clerks at the grocery stores would ask about Trude. Later, articles appeared in the local paper about my efforts to do something about Alzheimer's, and they made me even more recognized. People would stop me to tell me about a family member who suffered from the disease.

The suppositories were unfortunately necessary because Trude had lost the ability to move her bowels properly; the impulse we all have to do so when we are well had stopped functioning in her. She also had problems urinating, so I sometime had to use a catheter. I also had to keep track of her daily outputs because being unable to communicate and the frequent use of the catheter made bladder infections quite possible. I regularly checked her for bloating and wanted to make sure that she was not having internal problems that might cause her inexpressible pain.

I found different ways of occupying myself while I fed her. Sometimes I would stare out the window and watch the wind tear at the tree branches and watch the small grey winter birds scurry for cover or huddle down for warmth. Sometimes I reflect back on what our lives had been and sometimes I would sing along quietly to the old standards of Bennett, Miller, Dorsey and the like. Not many of our friends were as fortunate as Trude and I when it came to living it up, seeing the world and doing things. I had all of our adventures to rerun in my mind, and I could reflect on the good ol' days, and to quote Shakespeare, "…Call back yesterday, bid time return."

I fed her all of her meals myself. As difficult and distant as Trude now was, I still liked to spend time with her, and most of the people I hired didn't have the patience to spoon out the small bites required for her limited chewing and swallowing capabilities.

The long, slow process with the occasional pursed lips or refusal to eat reminded me of feeding the children when they were quite young, but with one key difference. When painstakingly feeding a child, there is the feeling that each day the child gets a little brighter and is more willing to assume part of the task of feeding himself (even if at first most of the food ends up on the face or the floor). While feeding Trude, there was the feeling that each day her light became a little dimmer. With the child is the certain hope that soon he will get to the point where this lengthy meal routine will no longer be necessary. With Trude there was the fear of what would happen when even spoon-feeding became impossible. It was hard not to get depressed during mealtime with the dark hovering on the horizon.

Nothing remained of her ability to eat, play, or even sleep as people routinely do. I fed her from a Gerber's dish that I kept warm with hot water—the kind one uses for a child. Her meat had to be put in a blender and her vegetables boiled to the point that they were soft enough to melt in her mouth—but also probably to the point that they had little nutritional value. The only sound during dinner was often me offering encouragement, such as, "Come on, dear, just a few more peas."

Even with Trude's loss of speech, I still would talk to her, and I hoped she knew what I was saying or that at least my voice provided some comfort. It's common for people with Alzheimer's to lose the ability to speak, but usually not as early as Trude did. Caring for her was a long, long day, made longer in Trude's case by the silence.

Rick would visit us regularly. He had always been extremely close to his mother, going back to his junior high days and their daily lunches. She was always there when he needed her, so now he wanted to be there for her, but it was so hard to tell what she needed. He had gotten in late one night after I had helped her into bed, so it was a surprise for her to see him that morning.

As I fed her breakfast, he walked into the room and she started to cry. Somewhere in the recesses of her mind she obviously knew this person was important to her, but being unable to place him must have been an awful torment for her. When he said, "It's me, Mom, Rick," all of us had tears in our eyes. When he spoke, she looked at him with an intensity that wasn't there for me, perhaps because she was immune to hearing my voice or perhaps because she was trying to remember who he was. It was like the horrible aftermath of a car accident—it was painful to stay and watch, but even harder to turn away.

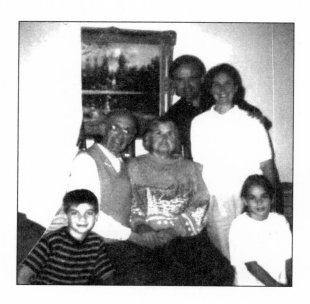

The whole family in
1996. Dave, me,
Trude, Rick, Judy and
Diana. (top)

Judy and Diana sit
with Trude.

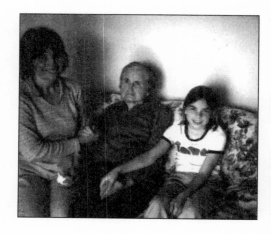

The Days Drag On

It became a common practice now that when Trude saw Judy or the grandchildren, she would cry. She must have felt the memories of them fading and it pained her deeply to be losing her offspring. Often Judy and Diana would sit next to Trude on the sofa, one on each side, with Diana usually holding Trude's hand. Trude seemed comforted by this. Perhaps it triggered fond memories of her motherly instinct toward our own children from long ago. Before they would leave for home, Diana would kiss Trude on the cheek and say with a soft but loving voice, "Bye-bye Grandma."

Trude was sick for so long that Diana had no clear memories of her grandmother that predated the glassy stare and rigid appearance that now characterized this once-beautiful woman. David had many fond memories of her from when he was small, but he sort of kept his distance now and seemed a bit uncomfortable around this hollow shell of a person. Could this be the same vibrant woman who swam with him in our pool?

These visits were draining on all of us, but it would have been sadder and lonelier for us all without them. Still, as close as we once were to the grandkids, one of the side effects of the disease was that we saw less of them now. It was hard to keep Trude in the car long enough to drive up to Wheeling, Illinois, to see them, and Trude's presence was clearly a bit unsettling to the kids. In my years of medical practice I had seen disease affect family members in different ways, some even afraid to touch someone with cancer as though they could catch it by contact. Trude's appearance was a bit "creepy" as David once described it.

In *Advances*, the Alzheimer's Association Newsletter, Edna L. Ballard was quoted as saying, "Caregivers grieve as they watch their spouses become shadows of their former selves. The most painful change brought about by this disease is the eventual disintegration of the characteristics and traits that previously defined the individual's personality and capacity for intimacy."

It very well summed up what I was feeling. I often wondered if Trude was alone in the darkness or if any of these visits or my presence meant anything to her.

It seemed destined that no matter where she was or who was caring for her, things would happen. I had tried to use the shower with her a few times, but that didn't work out very well, especially when she became flustered and frightened of what was about to happen, so I had started giving her sponge baths.

One morning after I had finished sponging her off, I started to lift her up from the portable chair next to the sink when she stepped forward haltingly from the carpet to the tile floor and her right foot went out from underneath her. She started to fall back, hitting the wall near the shower. She continued to slide toward the floor, and I reached out to try to slow her fall. But her momentum carried us both down, and we hit with a thump on the ledge of the shower stall. She cried a little, I thought as much from the fright as the pain. After regaining my own composure and footing, I cautiously helped her up not knowing if she had been injured. I carefully walked her to the bedroom so she could lie down while I examined her for bruises, cuts or other injuries. She appeared to be okay.

For most of the morning she rested on the sofa, and she seemed untroubled until I tried to raise her up. She winced terribly as I bent her forward. I stopped and tried a different way so as not to bend her spine at all. I had intended to feed her but instead called the ambulance to take her to the emergency room. Now the way she was reacting I was almost certain there was break in the spine so I asked to have an x-ray taken. I was afraid the fall might have caused the collapse of a bone or a complete break, but instead it showed a slight dent in the second bone of the lower part of her spine. Like many older women, Trude's bones had thinned.

We were able to go home the same day, and the doctor advised that for the next four to six weeks Trude should wear a back brace as much as possible. This seemed to offer some support and ease the pain a bit, but with an injury in the lower back, where so much bending and turning takes place, she was often in pain when she moved. There wasn't really much else that could be done, and I was just glad that she wasn't more seriously injured.

Alzheimer's had gradually but surely taken its toll on Trude's movements, which made her prone to topple over, so I just resolved to be more careful and not to assume she had her balance when we were moving.

As her stiffening got worse, I eventually had it investigated and an MRI showed this was Binswanger's disease, a neurological condition that describes the hardening of small arteries in the brain, which may cause the muscles to become inflexible and make movement even more difficult. The disease isn't related to Alzheimer's, nor is it caused by an injury; it just added to her problems. Walking became limited as her legs—first the right and then the left—became more affected. I would massage the muscles of her legs, but couldn't find a medication which would restore normal function. I tried having a physical therapist come to the house for a while, but that didn't help much, either.

I'd like to believe Trude's love for exercise delayed the progression of this disability and gave her a little added resistance, but I feared for the day when she would not be able to walk at all and wondered how I would move her if she could do nothing to move herself. I was never exactly robust, not even when I was unloading boxcars as a teenager, and now I found myself going on three-quarters of a century with more physical labor to do every day than I had done in 50 years. I tried to keep her walking rather than depend on a wheelchair all of the time, because I feared that her legs and then her circulation would go downhill even faster if she were even less mobile.

Standing her up was like lifting a wax statue since she would no longer bend at the waist. I would get both arms under hers and stand her up, then gently urge her forward, and she would walk as I soothingly said, "C'mon Baby, you can walk. Just one foot in front of the other." She had developed a habit of closing her eyes, and this made her even more likely to fall, so I had to stay with her to steady and steer her every step of the way.

Taking her to and from the table at mealtime, which hadn't been difficult a year before now, became a step-by-step balancing act to move 35 feet to the love seat or to the couch at the other end of the room. Getting her to and from the bedroom became a much more arduous journey as we did our awkward dance. I just tried not to rush things and would tell her I loved her as I helped her stumble along.

She would stand for a moment and then would slowly place a foot forward, but she had trouble placing her heel flat to the floor, so she would walk tippy-toed, which exaggerated her poor balance. At times she stumbled for a second but I would steady her and hold her closely. As we came into our bedroom, I helped her toward an old armchair, the same one that was in the breakfast room at the house in River Forest where she used to relax at the end of day. I would then dress her in a pajama top and a diaper. It saddened me that she now needed this embarrassing addition on a nightly basis. I'd help her to lie down on two pillows that I positioned to make her comfortable and I'd curl up against her.

After I'd got my arm underneath her neck, I would ask her for a goodnight kiss. She apparently still knew how, since after I kissed her forehead and her nose, sometimes she would pucker when I put my lips to hers. It still thrilled me to have her lips on mine and to have this last evidence that Trude was still with me. Certainly it wasn't quite as exciting as the night when she first French-kissed me in the back seat of the car, but made me very happy in a whole different way.

I feared for the day when Trude would fail to react at all and would lose one of the most important faculties, that we all need to live normally, the ability to give and receive love. Trude, the exceptional student, the secretary par excellence, artist, musician and a woman who could accomplish almost anything was soon to be relegated to a life of nothingness.

So often I felt she was in a suspended state or a realm where only she lived, staring into space without any reaction, and whether she knew I was there I couldn't tell until those rare moments like those kisses. It was not much, but made my day and gave me all the fulfillment I was to have. As George Bernard Shaw wrote, "love is a flame that is always burning itself out."

Later in 1996, after Trude and I had eaten and I had helped her to the couch, I noticed that she was quite warm and sweating. I took her pulse, blood pressure and temperature and decided something was wrong, so I took her to the hospital, and an EKG showed that she was having a heart attack. They kept her for four days until they were sure she was well enough to come home. I knew that no one in any care facility would have been paying close enough attention to notice the subtle changes that a small heart attack can produce.

That Christmas a strange thing happened. I was putting up a few decorations, nothing elaborate, but enough so that I wouldn't appear to be a complete Scrooge. I put on some Bing Crosby to try to put myself in the mood. When "White Christmas" came on, Trude suddenly brightened. She looked at the stereo expectantly and then looked back at me. For a moment I thought she was going to get off the couch and start dancing and singing. She clearly recognized the happiness that song represented. When the song was over, I played it again. It didn't happen. The moment had passed and the spell was broken. For months after that, I replayed that song once in a while and watched for some glimmer that it still touched her. Slowly I realized that no music would ever bring her back again and that I had seen her happy for the last time.

Studies are going on in many places to see if memories can be triggered by music. Often smiles, foot-tapping and finger drumming have been observed in patients who moments before were in far-off trances. I tried to play music with lyrics that I hoped might reach out to Trude through the haze. Even though Trude didn't like Frank Sinatra as a person, she never objected to his singing. One song that had a special meaning for us as young lovers was "Strangers in the Night."

Before she slid into a deeper Alzheimer's-imposed chasm, Trude had periods of apparent daydreaming that seemed more frequent and pleasant if familiar music was playing. I never disturbed those reveries and now it was sad that she no longer had even that escape.

The days just plodded along with all of 1997 a continuation of Trude's slow descent. The only highlight of the year was finally finding a good housekeeper, Bernadine Lewis, who stayed with us from then on. The nurse's aides still came and went faster than the change of seasons. As Trude became more helpless the burden placed on me and any other caregiver grew each day.

That year I also took her back to the Mayo Clinic to have her examined for abdominal pains, which turned out to be a bowel problem that had been present since her birth. They also confirmed so much of what I already knew concerning her Alzheimer's disease. Her arteries were hardening, which contributed to her stiffness and wasn't helping circulation to her brain.

When Rick visited these days, he would try hard to get her to smile or show any sign of recognition, but would leave feeling discouraged when he failed.

I spoke at an Alzheimer's conference put on by a health care company and we were all disappointed in the turnout. I guess until the disease hits close to home, it's hard for anyone to care.

The *Joliet Herald-News*, which years ago ran the photo that brought Trude and me together, did an article about my devotion to Trude that made me out to be some kind of a saint. I got lots of phone calls from patients telling me they would pray for us or asking for advice on their Alzheimer's problem. I thought if prayers could cure her, she would have been better long ago, with all the well-wishing I got.

A check-up in '98 revealed a kidney problem that required surgery, and from then on, Trude had to have a drainage tube running down to a bag strapped to her leg. I was concerned that she would tear at it or yank out the tube, but she never did. She somehow stayed patient during all of these tests and procedures, but the various ailments and her diminishing ability to eat were taking their toll and she was losing weight.

An old Sufi story tells of a group of animals lamenting the ways of humans, who are always taking from them. Each animal speaks up and tells the others the thing the humans take—eggs from the hen and milk from the cow. Then the snail speaks up, saying that he has something humans really want. And they'd take it too, if they could. But they can't because what the snail has is ... time.

I cherished the time I had remaining with Trude, because with her mounting illnesses I could see, all too clearly, we were running out of it.

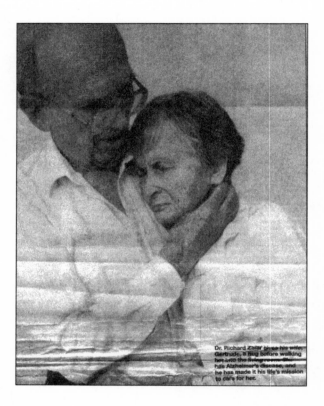

Dr. Richard Zatar hugs his wife Gertrude, a hug before walking her into the livingroom. She has Alzheimer's disease, and he has made it his life's mission to care for her.

The photo that appeared with the Chicago Tribune article about Trude and me with the caption, "Consuming love." *(photo by Tribune photographer John Smierciak)*

Rick helping his mother walk.

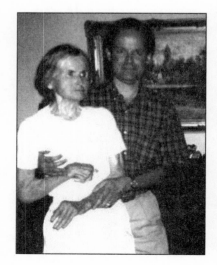

Last Hurrahs

My Christmas letter for 1999 gave an overview of the situation:

I have pretty much given up tending the yard, as it is a full-time job attending to Trude. The back yard is full of dandelions. I read the obit columns contain more and more familiar names.

Instead of a doctor, I am more frequently a patient now, on a host of pills. The diagnostic skills of most of the young physicians I am seeing leave much to be desired and I would have flunked them all if they had been my students at the Stritch School of Medicine.

Trude is in and out of the hospital a lot now with various problems including some trips to the ER. She is less than 100 pounds now and fading fast.

The new era of man in the new millennium is just ahead. At least I feel I quite humbly contributed some of my skill to helping others through the practice of medicine. Anything I have accomplished is thanks to my wonderful parents (although Momma died when I was three) who permitted me to grow and mature and to Trude—I would never have been able to sustain such an effort for 55 years without her by my side.

In the past few years we had still gone for our long walks, either in the nearby Louis Joliet Mall where many clerks in the stores would nod hello as we went by—or at a nearby river area, where our niece Mary Monica had a home. I'd park at her house while Trude and I took a stroll along the river, enjoying a touch of nature where we listened to the birds singing and swatched geese milling about on the large open plain near the water.

Most of our walks just took us around our neighborhood, and now it was only me walking and Trude riding in a wheel chair. I had to purchase a special one because as rigid as she was now—almost as straight as a board—she could slide out of the seat of a regular wheelchair. The new model had a reclining backrest and a safety belt to prevent that. She looked more comfortable this way. As she rode around the neighborhood, she didn't react at all as the neighbors said hello, instead just staring straight ahead, lost in her own world.

Probably all of our neighbors knew of Trude and me, since we were out so much. Often, as we passed, people would smile or ask, "How's the Missus?" or start a short conversation about the usual Illinois topic: the weather. It took us about a half-hour to make the four-block tour. When we arrived back at our home, if it was warm enough, I'd lock the wheels on the chair and face her toward the street while I got a chair from the garage for myself. We would sit there, and I would talk to her while I held her hand in mine. Now neighbors walking with their dogs or children would greet us. After a while, I'd wheel her up the wooden ramp and into the house.

One day as we reached the block behind our home and there were two young girls, about 8 or 9 years old, playing in the front yard of a home on the corner. I recognized the one of the girls from many of our other strolls, but didn't recognize the other, who must have been visiting. As we neared them, this girl said, "Hi. Is your mother sick? "

I replied, "Yes, she is, but she is my wife."

"Why does she just stare and look way out there?"

"She has an illness that won't let her talk or walk, and I can't get her well."

"Why don't you take her to a doctor? Maybe someone can make her better."

"I tried, but nothing has helped. Maybe someday when you girls are much older the doctors will have a cure or a shot, just like you had to have for measles and chickenpox so you didn't get sick. Wouldn't that be nice?"

She tried to smile some encouragement and waved goodbye.

As we headed home I thought about how much Trude loved children and would have enjoyed talking to them. I wished these girls could have known Trude when she was herself; they could have very much brightened one another's day.

On these walks I had too much time to reflect on what life had been. Author Joan Didion wrote something to the effect that we tell ourselves stories in order to live a life of fantasy at times. As I looked back on our lives, I thought of the many memorable and exciting occasions and appreciated what a good life we'd had. As I told myself the story of our lives, it all seemed rather perfect with none of the rough spots included. From the whole romance of our letters through watching the kids grow and prosper, there had to have been bad times, but I couldn't recall many. It seemed as though all of the bad times had waited to come at once.

As I pondered our last few years, I believed that fate had stepped in and dealt Trude a bad hand, but with a purpose. Our half-century of togetherness was more than I could have ever dreamed of, but I guess I never really appreciated it while it was going on. Too busy living our lives to stop and look at them.

Without Alzheimer's disease, how else would I have been able to discover so much about her? How else would I have been afforded this opportunity to support her in these trying days of her last illness? How else would I be able to enrich our love affair, as has been my good fortune during the last few years of her life? Most of our friends who are well enjoy each other in staid, repetitious lives and probably only peck each other on the cheek out of habit. Most of our married life, I'm now sorry to say, we lived by rote as well. I have a new appreciation for Trude because of what I have lost. I'm reminded of the line from a popular movie of our era, *Pride of the Yankees*, when Gary Cooper, as Lou Gehrig, stands before the crowd at Yankee Stadium and says as he is dying, "Today I am the luckiest man on the face of the earth." Sometimes I felt that way about the special time I had with Trude.

I bought a camcorder to try to preserve some memory of her. On the videos, she does nothing but stare, but I am glad I was able to capture some of her for later. I only wish I had a camera years ago, when she was still full of life and could have spoken and laughed.

Now more than ever, the days had a monotony and an unpredictability about them. Trude's worsening condition meant many trips to the hospital. Things would plod along in a set routine, only to be interrupted by various scares. It seemed odd for me to be seeing to her every need now, as she once so tenderly took care of me and the children.

I wrote to a friend:

Trude's not well and it is possible that she may end up in our local hospital. As I have mentioned in other letters or personal conversation, her physical status is becoming unpredictable. And I fear for her survival much longer. If she could just react to her infirmity (ies) so I could move in the right direction toward helping her. I am always guessing by objective manifestations and that isn't how a diagnosis is always confirmed.

The next few days will be critical in my life and in Trude's surely. It amazes me how the body and its structural elements can take such a beating day-in and day-out and still maintain a working order. I wish I could revitalize her to good health, but that is not to be.

Somehow we both survived that crisis, but I was running out of steam. Rick would caution me to try to take it easier, to let the nurse's aide do more, and I would grouse at him that no one cared anymore. When Russ Stevens stopped by, I would complain that I was exhausted and couldn't go on any longer and rant about the futility of it all, telling him I was going to end it all for Trude and myself. Usually by the next time I saw Russ I had forgotten that I had even told him I was at my wits' end. Russ was one of the few friends who consistently hung in there.

Many of our friends stopped coming around, and I couldn't say I blamed them. For those who had known Trude when she was vibrant and beautiful, to see her as the wasted shell of her former self was quite painful for them, as it was for me. At other times, I found myself getting angry at them and the rest of the world for abandoning me to my lonely plight.

Russ would stop by regularly and ask if I needed him to go to the store or anything. He always gave Trude a big friendly hello, even after it was apparent she wouldn't respond, and he always talked to both of us even though, again, it was obvious she wasn't really in the conversation. So many people just ignored her, as though she was a piece of furniture. Russ would let me prattle on about how much Trude enjoyed our walk or how we saw a flock of geese, knowing full well that it was unlikely she would have noticed a flock of 747s landing nearby, let alone a flock of birds.

I know I read emotions into her that she was no longer capable of feeling, but it made our walks and other activities more bearable to think she might be getting something out of them. I don't know how I would have coped if I thought there was really no point in doing any of the things I did for her. I'd probably have given up, and at some point perhaps I should have. Many people, including family and friends, would often say, "No one would blame you if you put her in a home." But I would have blamed me if anything else happened to add to her pain. And I did blame myself when she got hurt at the places I had chosen for her and for her falls while she was in my care.

In a story written about us in 1999 in the *Chicago Tribune*, the sub-headline read: "Retired doctor can do little to help his wife so he becomes her entire world and she becomes his." In the piece, Barbara Brotman wrote, "She is an echo of the woman he married, but he prefers the echo to silence." That was true.

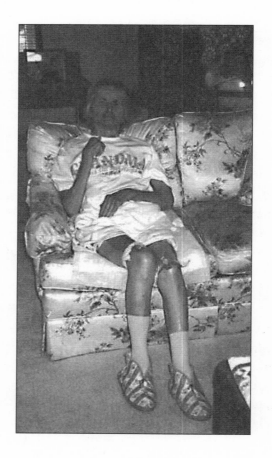

The state of Trude's sad condition by
late 1999. (top)

How Will it End?

Sometimes I would look at her and wonder how much Trude understood. Often her eyes were empty, vacant, staring blankly away at nothing and offering as little human connection as meeting the eyes of a department store mannequin. There was often less eye contact than one would find in a good painting by a master. Sometimes I would look at the sketch that was made of her in Paris and wish I could find in her living eyes as much life and energy as I saw in that portrait.

Every once in a while, certainly less frequently as the disease progressed, I could detect real recognition, real comprehension in her eyes. Somewhere, lost deep in the fog, something that was Trude still existed. I could do nothing but weep from fear that some part of her brain was still quite painfully aware of what had happened to the rest of her.

Occasionally, during the rare visits of someone outside the household, Trude would turn and look at them. Perhaps she was immune to the voices she heard every day, and something in a new voice would catch her attention. Often, when she did look at them, the eye contact was still lacking any sort of human touch, but once in a great while the visitor would report that they felt a genuine connection, a spark of recognition, like catching the eye of a stranger in a crowd and holding the eye contact so long that someone had to speak. Only Trude didn't. Couldn't. She quickly drifted off to whatever purgatory or hell held her most of the time.

In a book called *Alzheimer's Disease: A Guide for Families* by Lenore S. Powell with Katie Courtice, I found a passage that really struck home. I was confronted with similar questions without answers.

> *Whose life is it anyway; God's, the family's, society's, or the patient's? What if the patient is mentally incompetent? Why can't we help patients to die with dignity? Should the physician withhold treatment that seems to prolong the dying process when the patient will never regain the ability to make decisions and express his/her wishes? If the patient is conscious, does she/he have the right to tell the physician that she/he does not want cardiac resuscitation, tube feeding, or mechanical ventilation, or antibiotics? These questions become dilemmas in the face of society's moral and ethical repulsion toward suicide. The traditional tenet is that all human life is equally valuable. We must focus, however, on the quality of human life rather than the sanctity of human life. Is it humane or rational to preserve life when circumstances such as age or pain, or terminal illness suggest the burdens of life outweigh the benefits?*
>
> *What profits us to continue life in a vegetative state that can know no sound of music, no feel of wind, no smell of a rose, no memory of past loves, no feeling of present joy, but only pain, anguish, suffering and fear, with only more to look forward to each day. That is a living death, not life. Releasing the spirit of the Alzheimer's victim from the diseased brain is an act of human kindness. I believe that God will forgive this act and the soul will not suffer because of it.*

Each time I placed another depressing entry in the log I kept of Trude's condition, I was struck by how futile it was to let this go on. More than once I thought of what I might do to end her suffering.

Although caring for Trude was more than a full-time job, I did most of that caring in silence which gave me time—perhaps too much time—to consider my options.

Trude was dependent on a certified nurse-aide, a full-time housekeeper and me to keep her as comfortable and healthy as humanly possible. And through this all Trude was unable to express an opinion on so trivial a topic as what sort of soup she wanted, let alone her care or something as momentous as the ending of her life.

Several people had suggested that I just put her in a home and forget her, but after my experiences with even good facilities, I wasn't convinced that she could get proper and compassionate end-of-life care.

When some suggested Trude wouldn't know the difference, I protested that I would know the difference. So the question again became, was the life she was living with me worth living? While Trude was living at the French Center, I had spoken to their gero-psychiatrist about the wisdom of keeping someone alive with extraordinary measures after it was clear they were never coming back. We got no further than agreeing that it was pointless to use feeding tubes, respirators and machines for such people, Certainly neither the French Center's doctor nor I was advocating a wholesale euthanizing of patients, but he did add, "Now that we have found ways to lengthen people's lives, we owe it to those people to make their lives more comfortable." And, I would have added, safer.

I thought back on this discussion and how much easier it was to debate such topics in the abstract, before Trude was in such sad shape that I found myself even considering such things.

At what point is someone beyond hope? I knew Rick agreed with me that no major efforts should be made to keep his mother alive. The few times I had intervened, such as during her heart attack or kidney problem, without openly criticizing my judgment, he hinted that it might have been better to let one of those illnesses run its course rather than risk having his mother die of something even more painful and debilitating later.

Many Alzheimer's patients reach the point where they can't even remember how to swallow. It's not uncommon to put tubes down throats of people in comas to give them food and provide I.V. liquids to keep them alive until they recover consciousness. Most doctors won't do that with Alzheimer's cases, because there isn't much point in keeping them alive. For what? They aren't going to get better. And life can't be sustained indefinitely under those circumstances. Once it has been decided that you ethically, morally and lovingly can withhold nutrition and water and let someone die, is it that big a step to say life can be ended when it is no longer worth living?

I worried about how much Trude might be suffering. If any part of her brain was aware of what was happening to the rest of her, that had to be the worst kind of hell. To not even be able to scream in anguish as her life drifted away. So there were times when I resolved that the only humane thing to do was end her suffering. And I didn't want her to suffer even at the end, so I tried to think of the least painful ways: morphine or the car in the garage or maybe both. Sedate her and carry her to the car. This had the advantage that I could go with her.

There were other points to be considered. If Trude was gone, even without my help, would I want to live? If I somehow hastened her end, I was certain I would not.

In *Elegy for Iris*, John Bayley's book about his wife, he writes of a German professor who was part of the Oxford University faculty and was a good friend of Iris's. This professor had told close friends that when his terminally ill wife died, he would follow her, and he did by taking an overdose the same night she died. He knew the void left by her death would understandably be too much to bear. Bayley had asked himself the same question the professor and I had asked: was life worth living without a loving spouse?

So one of the problems with ending Trude's pain would be how to end my own afterwards.

If I did it, I would want to do it right. I would want to make sure there was enough gas in the tank. I would hate to wake up the next morning or have someone find me unconscious but alive. That would be embarrassing, and I'd hate to have to explain myself to the police or a court-appointed psychiatrist. A carbon monoxide overdose is painless and the dulling of the brain's responses and its activities are insidious but relentless until the final breath and the last heartbeat.

Someone close to me pointed out a good reason I couldn't do it. Not because of the moral aspects—he agreed that, at least in theory, Trude was better off dead and my logic of not wanting to live without her or to live to face the consequences was sound—but because of what this act would do to the rest of my family. He envisioned the headline, "Prominent Local Doctor in Murder-Suicide," and asked how big this news would be in this small town of Joliet, where many of mine and Trude's relatives still lived. I could cause huge problems for those I left behind, and my grandchildren were close enough to possibly suffer some fallout.

He suggested natural causes. Either letting one of Trude's many health problems go untreated or perhaps even helping things along a bit by leaving her outside on the deck for a while on a cold day. It sounded so cruel when stated that way, but was it any worse than slow starvation when she could no longer swallow at all? Was it more cruel than shoving a tube down the throat of someone who couldn't express a desire for it one way or the other?

There was another problem. Can anyone be certain that a person with even such a severe disability no longer wants to live? How could I be sure there wasn't some sort of satisfying fantasy life playing itself out in her mind?

Maybe there was some small patch of cells still striving to hold on. How could I presume to know about Trude? Although I studied her for some sign of something—some glimmer of light in her eyes—and found none, was there still a part of her that derived pleasure from my care and touch? Did some cluster of cells still get a thrill from hearing Rick's voice or Bing Crosby's or from Diana holding her hand or Judy kissing her cheek?

Even when a disease's path was much more clearly defined than Alzheimer's, I had never wanted to say for sure when a person was going to die, or presume to tell a family how they should handle certain critical decisions.

Deciding whether to remove feeding and hydration tubes, let alone actively ending someone's life, means also answering with brutal honesty the question, "Would I be doing it to end my loved one's suffering, or my own?"

The complications always made me stop and think. After too much thought I would always find myself reconsidering the whole idea. I never found the courage, if that's what it should be called, to hasten Trude's end.

Perhaps I made the more selfish choice. I wanted to preserve any time Trude had left, no matter what the cost to her or to me, and I dismissed any thoughts of helping Trude depart the black leather lounge seat in the family room forever. Even though I knew on one level that what was coming was what was best for Trude, I feared the inevitable more than I welcomed it.

I eventually stopped even entertaining thoughts and never quite decided if they were wise or foolish to begin with. As sad as the inevitable end was, I might be able to live afterwards. If I did anything to accelerate her fate, I knew there was no hope of that.

I read of a vile description by the wife of a man who had an advanced stage of Alzheimer's. She said it was, "Like being chained to a corpse." After I read it, I wondered how she could say that about a person she loved. She then tried to smooth out that harsh statement by adding, "Oh, a much-loved corpse," but the damage was done. I knew no matter what, my love for Trude would not die with her body's death, and her spirit would live with me forever.

James Thomas, who kept a diary of his life's daily happenings as he lost his faculties to Alzheimer's, noted:

> Most people expect to die someday, but who expected to lose their self first? I am hungry for the life that is being taken away from me. I am a human being. I still exist. I have a family. I hunger for friendship, happiness, and the touch of a loved hand. What I ask for is that what is left of my life shall have some meaning. Give me something to die for! Help me to be strong and free until my self no longer exists.

He also named his problem "God's cruel joke."

In my bitterness I submitted a Letter to the Editor of the *Herald News*, the same local daily that had brought us together in February 8, 1942. I titled it, "God is a mean old man." It was printed on the

editorial page under the heading, "Challenging the concept of God."
It read:

> The editorial page of this newspaper has been replete with articles
> regarding the presence of a God of the universe. In this brief interlude of
> meaningful interchange, I will reflect on those presentations and will proba-
> bly set the bibliophiles and the ministers of the faiths scurrying about to
> their mystic reference sources no doubt. And I do not want to eschew obfus-
> cation.
>
> If there is a God, a Deity, a Being, a Super-Force or whatever, and from
> what I have read and have heard from multiple sources, it is presumed, in
> an omniscient and omnipresent state, this Being exists in a Fatherly contin-
> uum. I really don't think this is absolute fact since no one has seen or heard
> from this Personage (not even Moses and the Burning Bush episode is gospel
> true. Who was there?)
>
> And I challenge the FATHER concept and all that implies for as a parent
> myself, which portends responsibility and so much more, I find this God,
> lacking. HE created us, an image of HIS likeness, and the complex and
> unbelievably incomprehensible basic structure of the organism, known as
> the human species is HIS work. This means the DNA, RNA, and their
> cogeners and the thousands of genes presently under investigative study
> were HIS idea and by skillful planning, a composite picture resulted. Now, if
> this is not so, then the evolutionists gain respect immediately. With these
> facts in hand I seek an answer.
>
> In a more specific sense, and because I am considerate of all, especially
> when my children and my daughter's children, are involved, a question arises.
> If the above set of scientific methodologies and chemical events are so factual,
> then how could this GOD permit any human being to be programmed from
> the time of the egg and sperm interaction until death intervenes progressing to
> a complete degradation of the spirit and the body as is occurring in many of
> us, (including foremost, my wife, Trude). I surely wouldn't want my children
> to suffer, if I had a say-so in their coding of life's events.
>
> I know if I had such power I wouldn't build my product to agonize, to
> endure unbearable ignominy, that would be cruelty beyond belief and mean-
> ness that belies description. And if this BEING, this GOD, this ENTITY,
> this SUPER-FORCE is still around, or was ever involved, then there is a

*touch of sadism here at the worst. In that case, HE must have a grudge
against all of MANKIND, and for sure, is a mean old man.*

*And please don't tell me the struggle with this form of life's travails is a
cross to bear and the ticket to the heavenly choirs or something akin. I
haven't talked to anyone lately who has been there to prove that point. This
is not blasphemy either but simple logic of the day.*

Within a few days, responses filled the editorial page of the paper
with headings such as: "God doesn't have a grudge against mankind,"
"A tragedy causes people to question God," "Why doesn't God just
make a perfect world," "God lacks nothing; we are the ones lacking,"
"Strength to go on," and "He trampled on the spirituality of others."

One helpful and sympathetic response came from a man named
Jack Miles, who wrote:

*I should begin by saying that I am sorry for the loss you are suffering in
seeing your wife disappear into Alzheimer's disease. I know that in so many
ways, this seems worse than death. Such suffering, such disintegration seems
completely pointless and completely incompatible with the notion that God
is both fatherly in spirit and all-powerful. I myself do not claim to know
whether God exists. I have a keen sense of the likely limitations of the
human mind, and therefore have no great confidence that science understands the world or even has a reliable method or framework for understanding it. But the comfort that may be there in the notion that the world is ulti-
mately mysterious is a pretty cold comfort. We may take God to be the
character who stars in the Bible. We may also take the word god to be a
name for our inability ever fully to understand what is happening to us.*

Once I decided to finish the story as if some unseen hand had written it, I decided to seek the assistance of the local hospice. I had heard
from old patients how much the caring compassion of the hospice
volunteers helped ease the transition. They were used to dealing with
a lot of details that are difficult to face at such a trying time. I set an
appointment for a nurse and social worker to come to the house.

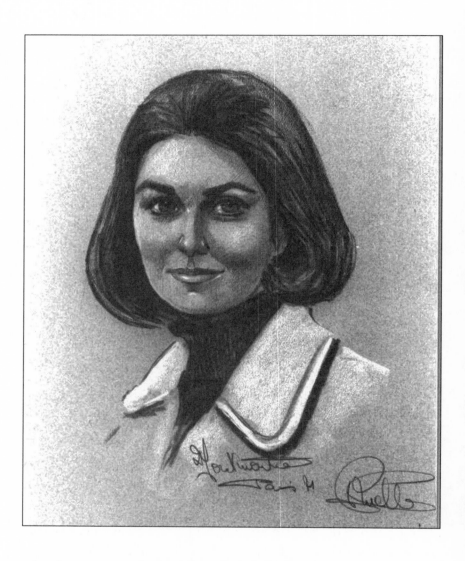

The charcoal sketch of Trude done in Paris.

Time to Say Goodbye

D ecember 7, 2000, was gray and overcast. That morning, snow was scattered here and there, barely covering the grass and just dusting the barren poplar trees that stand as five sentinels across our back yard. In the Midwest, and especially where we live, in a snow belt south of Chicago, we seem to be at the mercy of nature so anything can happen. The early appearance of snow had kept Trude in the house since her overall condition was so poor it wasn't good for her to go out, and it was hard to push the wheelchair in the snow. She hadn't been out for months. I always thought she looked and felt better after a short trip here or there, so the lack of outdoor exposure had her looking even more pale and sickly.

I had been expecting the end for so long that when it finally came, it took me completely by surprise.

I opened the blinds to admit what little light was filtering down through the clouds. It was seven o'clock, and the dreariness of the bleak and leaden skies wasn't very encouraging. Rain had fallen during the night, and the porch deck had puddles, but at least there wasn't any snow.

I went through my usual morning ritual of dressing and shaving and finished about seven-thirty. I then sat down in the black recliner next to our bed. I closed my eyes for a moment to wait for her to make a move, showing me she was awake. A few moments later I noticed a change in her facial expression—a sort of grimace, as though she might be in pain. I waited and spoke to her gently, stroking the side of her face.

"C'mon, Baby Dear, it's time to get breakfast. Let me rub your legs first."

I always rubbed her thin and weakened legs, just to get the blood moving before I would have her try to stand. Then, I would sit her at the edge of the bed, lifting her up by holding her in my arms so she didn't fall. This morning, something didn't seem quite right with her, but I lifted her into the lounge chair three feet away and let her down into the soft, black, leathered seat. I had gotten used to her blank eyes, but this morning the way she stared was even more vacant.

After I got her breakfast ready, I spooned a small amount of water into her mouth, and waited to see if she would swallow it. Her intake of any kind of liquid had not been good lately. Even the tea that she would always have with lunch held no interest for her. I noticed swallowing these days was more difficult. She still hadn't swallowed the water, and she seemed to be in a trance, even further away from things than usual. When it was apparent this phase not going to pass anytime soon, I thought it better for her to be back in bed.

She appeared even weaker and less responsive than was now the norm for her condition.

I picked her up in my arms and laid her down on her side of the bed, snuggling her head on two pillows. I laid down beside her with her head in the crook of my left arm. She kept staring ahead, and her mouth was partially opened. I talked to her as I caressed her face, but she didn't react at all.

Her breathing was also changing, from deep sighs to times when I could barely see any movement of her chest. I became frightened. I asked softly, "Darling, please wake up for me." I kissed her cheek; rubbed her arms and asked again, "Baby doll, c'mon, try to look at me. Wake up so we can eat our breakfast."

I checked her wrists for a pulse, but her injured right forearm made it difficult to detect a beat, so I tried the left. There was just a faint thump against my finger. I tried to awaken her again but nothing happened. "Sweetheart, wake up. Open your eyes."

My heart sank. Something was dreadfully wrong. I rested my hand on her stomach and breathed a sigh of relief when I got a good pulse there. She was still breathing erratically, so I checked her mouth. Lately she had been swallowing so poorly, I thought she might have some food stuck in her throat from a day or two ago, although she had had no problem last night, as had happened during dinner a couple of times during the past week. Then she had started to make little choking sounds in her throat, as if she couldn't swallow, even though the portions were very small and very soft. Now, her breathing became labored and she gave a weak cough a few times.

I noticed a changing motion of her chest. It seemed normal for a bit. Then it was difficult to see any movement, and a slight gurgling sound would come and go. I hoped this meant she would be coming out of her trance-like state soon. She had had other spells like this, but none that lasted as long or that felt so disconcerting. I glanced at the clock on the dresser which read 10:30. I had been trying to wake her for over an hour.

Suddenly, she seemed to swallow noisily, with a choking sound, and then quieted. I didn't see her chest move, and I put my hand on her stomach area trying to find the thump I had just felt. It was gone! I couldn't believe it.

I pleaded, "Sweetheart, don't leave me! Don't leave me! Baby-Dear, come on now, breathe! Please, Baby-Dear. Can you hear me?" The tears were choking my words as I implored her to hang on.

I called to the housekeeper and nurse-aide who were in the kitchen just outside the bedroom: "Roseanne! Bernadine! Come here. Trude's gone! I can't do anything about it!"

I cried and cried and cried. She had died quietly and without pain, as far as I could tell. I kept holding her in my arms like I always did and kept talking to her. She understood, I'm sure. About a half-hour later, hospice staff arrived, and the nurse took over. I had spoken to the service a week earlier asking for assistance, and today was to have been their first visit. It was, but at the wrong time and for the wrong purpose. I went to the other bedroom, absolutely beside myself and not knowing where to go or what to do next.

Trude was dead, and I was alone for the first time in 58 years. After a while, Roseanne came to the door and asked if she could do anything. I asked her to call Rick and Judy and tell them what happened to their mother. I couldn't do it.

I cried quite a bit after she was gone. Anytime I thought of her. And anything could make me think of her. Day or night. Snow or rain. It didn't make a lot of difference. It took a long time for the tears to wash my soul. I expected to have some cathartic moment when suddenly the pall lifted. It didn't happen. She still moves through every room and through every minute of every day. I feel the void, and it's immeasurable. What should I do? I thought once again about going to the garage and, with its door tightly closed, getting into the car and starting the engine. As I see it, suicide is an act of desperation or satisfaction, nothing more, nothing less. I wasn't that desperate and didn't know what I would satisfy in doing it.

Strangely, December 7 was a date which, for so many, set their lives on a course of tragedy and loss, for others meant their lives were sent off in a direction that would bring opportunity, travel, adventure, and in some cases, romance. A minor, minor side effect of the events set in motion that day changed my life in a way that at age 19 I couldn't have dreamed possible.

Ironically, 59 years later, it was another December 7 that would fill me with a sense of loss and make me curse that day as most others of my generation have since 1941. My first contact with Trude was prompted by a photo published because of the war. If the war had not begun, she would not have had her photo in the paper and this romance would never have happened and my life would have been immeasurably different and undoubtedly poorer.

I got many cards and notes, but one from my niece especially touched and seemed to sum up what I was feeling:

Dear Uncle Dick,

After leaving Joliet I was away a few days. Upon my return, a message from Betsy advised me about Aunt Trude. Uncle Dick I am so terribly sorry. You two shared a great love. Your devotion seemed boundless and I have never seen its like. It seems only poets and composers shared that kind of love with you and Aunt Trude.

I tried to find an appropriate card but none seemed to quite suit her. When I think of Aunt Trude I see bright, cheerful colors, her eyes so large and expressive, shining dark hair that swayed and moved when she did, a smile so grand it seemed to fill the room, a musical lyrical voice and laugh— there was something about her that just seemed glowing and it warmed you. How could anyone not love her? But no one could love her like you do. I know words mean very little but I wanted you to know my thoughts.

May it comfort you to remember always that you surrounded Aunt Trude with love and she knew it...I'm sure.

Love, Mary

I still have trouble accepting what this illness took from her and from me, both before and after she died. As Judy once said, it was as though her mother died twice. Once, when she ceased to have any resemblance to the lively, wonderful mother she was, and then again, when her body finally gave out.

Rick said she probably lived at least six months longer than she should have. He said no one would have taken the time to painstakingly feed her the way I did, and we had agreed there would be no feeding tube when she could no longer eat on her own. There was no point in calling an ambulance for her that last day. Any superhuman efforts that might have brought her back would have done so only temporarily.

I visit the cemetery every day I can. It makes me feel closer to her somehow. I had our code—the Gregg shorthand squiggles for "P.S. I love you very much, always will, remember," etched on her gravestone. I have had people ask me if it is Arabic or some eastern European language.

Ever since our first date and until close to the end, when her illness took so much away from her, there was something in the way she moved that attracted me. I cannot describe it in just so many words but I saw it. Love acts in strange ways. Why do we find some people attractive and not others? From the first moment I saw her photo in the paper I was drawn to her. Whenever I thought of her smile, I knew I didn't need another lover, ever, and was never the least bit tempted to look elsewhere. I'm sure I could never again find what I had with Trude, even if I were looking.

I still get phone calls from former patients wanting medical advice or from people who have read about me in the paper and want to know what to do with a family member or friend who seems to have Alzheimer's. I wish I had an answer. I offer what words of encouragement I can, but shudder when I think of what a long and sad journey they have begun.

Many mornings I sit in the chair next to our bed, looking at the charcoal sketches tacked to the wall. Trude did those 40 years ago, but they still look as fresh and new as today's weather. The drawing of her seems more real to me than her photos, I guess because it was done by her hand, and therefore is a part of her. It also helps keep me close to my memories of my girl, Trude.

In any story written with an ending that is known from the start or at least pre-supposed, it's always nice to find a bit of good to remember, so I like to think back to our first kiss after the senior prom at the University of Illinois on May 25, 1942.

Crying does me some good now, but I still miss her and I'm sure the loneliness will never go away. I take solace in the fact that given my age and health, I shall be with her soon, I am sure.

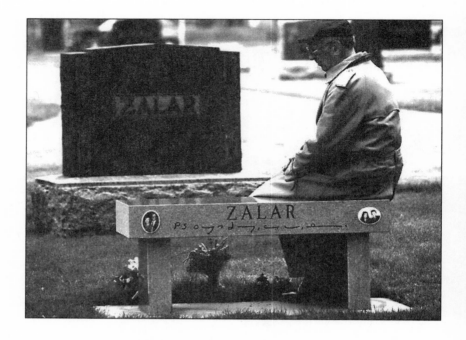

Me at Trude's grave. Inscribed on the bench is our shorthand code.

Afternoon in February

by Henry Wadsworth Longfellow

The day is ending,
The night is descending;
The marsh is frozen,
The river dead.
Through clouds like ashes
The red sun flashes
On village windows
That glimmer red.
The snow recommences;
The buried fences
Mark no longer
The road o'er the plain;
While through the meadows,
Like fearful shadows,
Slowly passes
A funeral train.
The bell is pealing,
And every feeling
Within me responds
To the dismal knell;
Shadows are trailing,
My heart is bewailing
And tolling within
Like a funeral bell.

Wednesday
3/3/43

Dearest Darling,

Just couldn't go to bed without first writing to you & telling you that I had a perfect evening being with you. Enjoyed it very much & being with you is superb. Hated to see you go, sweetie, and I'm very happy that I thought of the telephone nook as a place to kiss you goodnight. It certainly would have been a calamity if you'd have gone without a few real goodnight kisses. For two so in love, goodnight kisses are a must, and without them we would feel a bit on the sad and blue side. Right?

Afterword

The letters reproduced in this book are actual transcriptions of some of the correspondence Trude and I wrote. They have been kept pretty much intact as they were written so typos, spelling and punctuation have been preserved. I apologize to those whose names were wrongly spelled, including Garland McCowan (Cramer), whose name Trude misspelled in her original letter, but I did not want to tamper with the text of the letters, so that they could be read as they were written. Some have been shortened with irrelevant parts dropped.

The long love affair I had with Trude was not ended by her death. Our son once said that since I failed to preserve her life I seem determined to preserve her memory. Maybe that is what motivated me to write this book and to make sure her name lives on in various ways.

I have endowed an annual award at our alma mater, Joliet Township High School, in her name for the girl in each graduating class who has the highest grade-point average.

I provided funds for a lecture series about Alzheimer's disease at the Stritch School of Medicine at Loyola University.

Through the John Douglas French Center in Los Alamitos, California, I donated money for the "Caring Touch Award," which gives a prize to a caregiver of the year.

Most of my time is now spent trying to fund and build a model care facility specially designed for Alzheimer's patients to be built on land in Joliet generously donated by a thoughtful local family.

Tax-deductible* donations to the Gertrude P. Zalar Alzheimer Care Foundation may be made by sending a check to:
GERTRUDE P. ZALAR ALZHEIMER CARE FOUNDATION
1081 CHOVAN DRIVE
JOLIET, IL 60435

www.gpzalarfoundation.com

email: info@GPzalarfoundation.com

Additional copies of this book may be obtained through the Foundation, with discounts available to qualifying groups.

Thank you for taking the time to share my story and perhaps, with your help, others will be spared the ravages of this disease.

* The Gertrude P. Zalar Azheimer Care Foundation is a 501 (e)(3) entity under provisions of the IRS code.

Acknowledgements

This project would not have been possible without the help of many people. First, as far as the book itself I would like to thank:

Walt Meyer, who "forced" me to develop a mission statement and took my assemblage of words, phrases, ideas, thoughts, and musings, and created something from the heart. Walter is a taskmaster, to be sure, and that's why he has been successful in what he does best—writing.

Ann Smolen for looking over the manuscript and catching errors.

Likewise, Mr. and Mrs. Gilbert Meyer for reviewing the text and making suggestions.

The Mavericks writer's group for their insightful comments.

Novelist Martin J. Smith for putting me in contact with Mr. Meyer.

Richard E. Cheverton for turning this manuscript into a book.

For information on Alzheimer's disease, I am indebted to:

Ferri Kidane, former executive director of the John Douglas French Center in Los Alamitos, California.

For help with the story itself, I must thank:

Russ Stevens for his friendship for more than 60 years, as well for the information he provided for this manuscript.

Trude's and my children, Dr. Richard W. Zalar, Jr. and Barbara Judy Wesoloski, and her children, Dave and Diana, and their father, Ron Wesoloski, for their input on the book as well as their love and support.

About the authors:

RICHARD WAYNE ZALAR, SR. is a retired physician whose specialty was internal medicine. He still regularly gets phone calls from his former patients wanting his advice. He served in the Army Medical Corps during and just after World War II, leaving the service with the rank of captain in 1947. Besides practicing medicine in the Chicago area and in Southern California, Dr. Zalar taught at the Chicago Medical School, the University of Illinois Medical School, Cook County Graduate School, and the Stritch School of Medicine at Loyola University. He has been published in numerous medical journals including the American Journal of Digestive Disorders. He was recognized by the Chicago Medical Society for 50 years of medicine.

Like his late wife, Richard Zalar, Sr. was born in Joliet, Illinois and lived in the Chicago area most of his life. Trude and Dick were married in 1944, and they raised two children, Dr. Richard W. Zalar, Jr. and Barbara Judy Wesoloski, and have two grandchildren, David and Diana Wesoloski.

In 1993, Dr. Zalar retired from his medical practice to devote himself full-time to his wife's care after Trude became seriously ill with Alzheimer's disease. Trude died in December 2000. Their story gained national attention through a series of articles, including one in the *Chicago Tribune*.

Dr. Zalar now devotes his time to the Gertrude P. Zalar Alzheimer Care Foundation, which he established in her memory to help care for victims of this disease until a cure or treatment is found, and to the Zalar Center of Excellence Corporation that will be instrumental in the construction and medical control of the Gertrude P. Zalar Alzheimer Management Center—a state of the art care facility—which is to be built in Illinois.

WALTER G. MEYER is a free-lance writer based in San Diego. Born and raised in the suburbs of Pittsburgh, he always knew he wanted to be a writer, and this desire was reinforced when, in the 4th grade, he won a short-story contest sponsored by *The Atlantic Monthly*. He wrote for his elementary school paper, his high school newspaper (turning "pro" in the 9th grade by selling his first paid work to the local news-

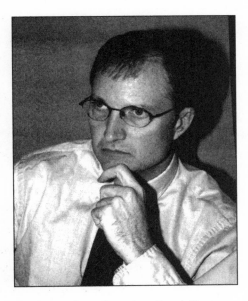

paper), then going on to write for *The Daily Collegian* at Penn State.

He has written for numerous newspapers and magazines including *Kiplinger's Personal Finance, Los Angeles Times Magazine, The Orange County Register, The (Portland) Oregonian, Out, Pittsburgh Press*, among many others.

Mr. Meyer has written everything from a comic strip and greeting cards to screenplays and books. His most recent book, *Going for the Green: Selling in the 21st Century*, a business how-to book written in the form of a novel, was published in 2001. He is not related to any of the people named Meyer mentioned in the book.